Novel Biomaterials for Tissue Engineering

Edited by Petrica Vizureanu and Madalina Simona Baltatu

Published in London, United Kingdom

Novel Biomaterials for Tissue Engineering
http://dx.doi.org/10.5772/intechopen.110991
Edited by Petrica Vizureanu and Madalina Simona Baltatu

Contributors
Aby Mathew T, Alenya Mary Pyas, Andrei Victor Sandu, Annie Thomas, Aswathy S, Chamalayil AbdulRahman Syed Mohammed Jiffry, Chiamaka Okafor, Derick Joseph, Mathew John, Farida ElGamal, G. Meenu, Jerin Thomas, Johnson Dlima, Jose Paul, Kavya Suresh, Lekshmi Mini, Madalina Simona Baltatu, Mekha Grace Varghese, Mihaela Claudia Spataru, Nebu G. George Thomas, Nibu Varghese, Norman Munroe, Petrica Vizureanu, Prameetha George Ittycheria, Puthiya Veettil Darshana, Rakhi Manohar, Rene Kuriakose, Rupesh S, Sajith Vellapally, Sameer KM, Saumya John, Senny Thomas Parackal, Sruthi K. Nair, Valliaveettil Thomas George, Vimal Thomas

First published in London, United Kingdom, 2024 by IntechOpen
IntechOpen is the global imprint of INTECHOPEN LIMITED, registered in England and Wales, registration number: 11086078, 167-169 Great Portland Street, London, W1W 5PF, United Kingdom

British Library Cataloguing-in-Publication Data
A catalogue record for this book is available from the British Library

Additional hard and PDF copies can be obtained from orders@intechopen.com

Novel Biomaterials for Tissue Engineering
Edited by Petrica Vizureanu and Madalina Simona Baltatu
p. cm.

This title is part of the Biomedical Engineering Book Series, Volume 23
Topic: Biotechnology - Biosensors, Biomaterials and Tissue Engineering
Series Editor: Robert Koprowski
Topic Editor: Luis Jesús Villarreal-Gómez

Print ISBN 978-1-83769-228-6
Online ISBN 978-1-83769-229-3
eBook (PDF) ISBN 978-1-83769-230-9
ISSN 2631-5343

For EU product safety concerns:
IN TECH d.o.o., Prolaz Marije Krucifikse Kozulić 3, 51000 Rijeka, Croatia,
info@intechopen.com or visit our website at intechopen.com.

IntechOpen Book Series

Biomedical Engineering

Volume 23

Aims and Scope of the Series

Biomedical Engineering is one of the fastest-growing interdisciplinary branches of science and industry. The combination of electronics and computer science with biology and medicine has improved patient diagnosis, reduced rehabilitation time, and helped to facilitate a better quality of life. Nowadays, all medical imaging devices, medical instruments, or new laboratory techniques result from the cooperation of specialists in various fields. The series of Biomedical Engineering books covers such areas of knowledge as chemistry, physics, electronics, medicine, and biology. This series is intended for doctors, engineers, and scientists involved in biomedical engineering or those wanting to start working in this field.

Meet the Series Editor

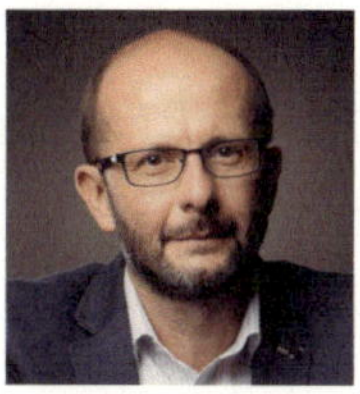

Robert Koprowski, MD (1997), Ph.D. (2003), Habilitation (2015), is an employee of the University of Silesia, Poland, Institute of Computer Science, Department of Biomedical Computer Systems. For 20 years, he has studied the analysis and processing of biomedical images, emphasizing the full automation of measurement for a large inter-individual variability of patients. Dr. Koprowski has authored more than a hundred research papers with dozens in impact factor (IF) journals and has authored or co-authored six books. Additionally, he is the author of several national and international patents in the field of biomedical devices and imaging. Since 2011, he has been a reviewer of grants and projects (including EU projects) in biomedical engineering.

Meet the Volume Editors

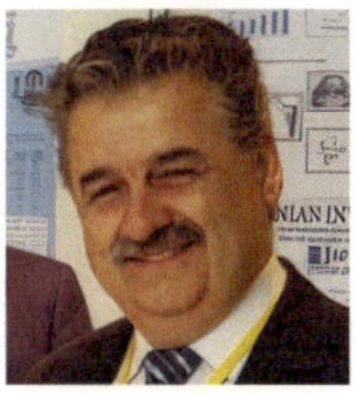

Petrica Vizureanu obtained an MSc and Ph.D. in Heating Equipment at the "Gheorghe Asachi" Technical University, Iasi, Romania, in 1992 and 1999, respectively. Dr. Vizureanu is currently a full professor and scientific supervisor in materials engineering at the same university and the appointed director of the Department of Technologies and Equipment for Materials Processing. He is an editor and guest editor for many journals and publishing houses. His research focuses on expert systems for heating system programming, computer-assisted design for heating equipment, heating equipment for materials processing, heat transfer, biomaterials, and geopolymers. He has published more than 250 papers in international journals/conference proceedings and more than 40 books.

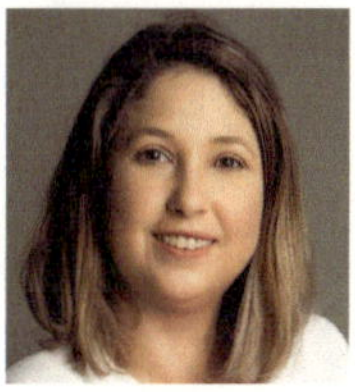

Madalina Simona Baltatu is a lecturer at the "Gheorghe Asachi" Technical University, Iasi, Romania. She obtained her Ph.D. in 2017. She is a researcher with experience in biomaterials. She has published 6 books, 4 book chapters, and 60 journal and conference papers. She also has five patent applications to her credit. Dr. Bălțatu is the recipient of 56 awards obtained at invention salons (32 gold medals, 7 silver medals, 2 bronze medals, 15 special awards).

Contents

Preface

Novel Biomaterials for Tissue Engineering provides an overview of the trends in biomaterials used in tissue engineering, addressing numerous innovative materials that can be integrated into future medical applications. This book is the result of society's need for new materials and trends in medicine due to increasingly complex challenges, as well as the need for sustainable and efficient solutions. The book comprises eight chapters and is structured into two sections: "Novel Biomaterials" and "Trends in Tissue Engineering."

In the first section, "Novel Biomaterials", the book explores the general trends in the application of biomaterials, highlighting both their advantages and limitations in various medical fields. It discusses the importance of selecting and designing biomaterials based on the specific requirements of medical applications, considering biocompatibility, mechanical properties, wear and corrosion resistance, and osseointegration.

The second section, "Trends on Tissue Engineering", continues with a discussion on nanofibers for skin regeneration and wound treatment applications, followed by an analysis of manufacturing techniques for scaffolds applied in regenerative medicine. This section emphasizes the essential role of scaffolds in providing a three-dimensional environment for tissue regeneration and discusses various manufacturing methods, from conventional to advanced techniques such as 3D bioprinting.

In conclusion, the book offers a comprehensive perspective on the role of new biomaterials in tissue engineering and regenerative medicine, highlighting significant progress, current challenges, and future research directions in this dynamic field. We thank all national and international authors for their excellent contribution, which has significantly enriched our study field.

We hope this book proves to be a valuable source of inspiration for researchers, biomaterials engineers, students, and medical professionals, offering an in-depth exploration of the latest discoveries and emerging technologies in the manufacturing of innovative biomaterials.

Petrica Vizureanu and Madalina Simona Baltatu
Faculty of Materials Science and Engineering,
Gheorghe Asachi Technical University of Iasi,
Iasi, Romania

Section 1

Novel Biomaterials

Chapter 1

General Trends on Biomaterials Applications: Advantages and Limitations

Mihaela Claudia Spataru, Madalina Simona Baltatu, Andrei Victor Sandu and Petrica Vizureanu

Abstract

The field of biomaterials has witnessed significant advancements in recent years, with increasing applications in various medical disciplines. This book chapter provides an overview of the trends in biomaterials applications, highlighting their advantages and limitations. Biomaterials play a critical role in improving patient outcomes, enabling the development of innovative medical devices, and enhancing the quality of life. They find extensive use in orthopedics, esthetic surgery, ophthalmology, maxillofacial surgery, cardiology, urology, neurology, and other medical specialties. While biomaterials offer numerous benefits, their selection and design depend on specific medical applications. Biocompatibility, adequate mechanical properties, physical and chemical characteristics, wear resistance, corrosion resistance, and osseointegration are important considerations. However, the complexity of the biological environment and the lack of detailed knowledge about in vivo conditions pose challenges. The success of an implant replacement relies on the tissue-material interface, which varies based on the desired outcome. Hemocompatible behavior is necessary for implants in contact with blood, whereas osseointegrated implants require a strong interaction for high adhesion force. This chapter also discusses the limitations of biomaterials, including immune reactions, limited biocompatibility, durability issues, interactions with the surrounding environment, lack of regeneration, high costs, and design constraints. It emphasizes the importance of ongoing research and development to overcome these limitations and advance the field of biomaterials.

Keywords: biomaterials, classification, medical applications, advantages, limitations

1. Introduction

Biomaterials are constantly used in the medical field and can be defined as "materials that present new properties that make them suitable to come into direct contact with living tissue without causing an immune rejection or an adverse reaction" [1]. It should be mentioned that the prefix "bio" of biomaterials refers to "biocompatible," rather than "biological" or "biomedical," as is often misinterpreted [2–5].

Biomaterials have been utilized in various forms throughout antiquity, demonstrating the ingenuity and resourcefulness of ancient civilizations. Although the concept of biomaterials as we understand them today was not fully developed, ancient societies intuitively utilized natural materials with desirable properties for medical purposes. In ancient Egypt, linen and papyrus were employed as bandages and wound dressings, providing protection and aiding in healing [6, 7]. Natural resins like myrrh and frankincense, known for their antimicrobial properties, were incorporated into ointments and balms. In ancient Greece, honey was used for its antibacterial and anti-inflammatory effects, while olive oil served as a moisturizer and enhancer of medicinal herbs. Traditional Chinese medicine relied on biomaterials derived from plants, animals, and minerals. Herbal remedies with ginseng, *aloe vera*, and pearl powder promoted healing and rejuvenation. Natural substances like shells, bones, and stones were used for their mechanical properties in bone setting and acupuncture. These early practices laid the foundation for the development of modern biomaterials in medicine [8–11].

The first generation of biomaterials emerged in the 1950s and 1960s and primarily consisted of industrial materials that were not specifically developed for medical use. These biomaterials were selected based on their physical properties relevant to the intended clinical application and their bioinert nature, meaning they elicited minimal response in host tissues and were considered biocompatible. Common materials included polymers, metals, and ceramics. The primary goal of first-generation biomaterials was to achieve an appropriate combination of functional properties that matched the replaced tissue without eliciting deleterious host responses. Examples of first-generation biomaterials include pyrolytic carbon, initially developed for coating nuclear fuel particles, and later used in modified forms to coat mechanical heart valve components [12–14].

The second generation of biomaterials evolved from the first generation and aimed to induce specific therapeutic effects by causing controlled reactions with the surrounding tissues. These bioactive materials were designed to interact with the host tissue to achieve desired outcomes [14–16]. Examples of second-generation biomaterials include bioactive glasses and ceramics used in orthopedic and dental surgeries for localized controlled drug release applications. Another example is the HeartMate® left ventricular assist device, which features a textured polyurethane surface that promotes a controlled thrombotic reaction to minimize the risk of blood clotting. Drug-eluting endovascular stents, which limit restenosis (blood vessel closure) after balloon angioplasty, are also considered second-generation biomaterials [17–19].

Additionally, the second generation saw the development of resorbable biomaterials that could be degraded over time. These biomaterials had tailored degradation rates, allowing them to be absorbed by the host tissue and eliminating the need for long-term foreign materials. A well-known example is the use of biodegradable sutures composed of polyglycolic acid (PGA) since the 1960s. Ongoing research focuses on finding biodegradable polymers with properties such as strength, flexibility, tissue-friendly composition, and degradation rates suitable for specific applications. Novel properties like shape memory and programmable and interactive surfaces controlling the cellular microenvironment are also being investigated within the realm of second-generation biomaterials [20].

Biomaterials play an essential role in the human body by serving as artificial substitutes or implants that interact with living tissues, organs, and bodily fluids. They contribute to various medical treatments, therapies, and interventions, improving patient health and quality of life. In **Table 1.** are the essential roles of biomaterials in the human body [21–23].

Application	Description	Example
Medical Implants	Biomaterials are used as implants to replace or support damaged or dysfunctional body parts	joint replacements, heart valves, pacemakers, and vascular stents, restoring cardiovascular functionality
Tissue Engineering and Regenerative Medicine	Play an important role in tissue engineering and regenerative medicine. They provide scaffolds or matrices to support the growth and regeneration of tissues and organs. These biomaterial scaffolds mimic the extracellular environment and guide cell growth, leading to the formation of new tissue	skin grafts, bone grafts, and artificial organs
Drug Delivery Systems	Are used as carriers or vehicles for controlled drug delivery. They can be engineered to release drugs or therapeutic agents in a controlled manner, targeting specific tissues or cells. This approach improves drug efficacy, reduces side effects, and enhances patient compliance	Implants, nanoparticles, hydrogels, or microparticles
Diagnostic and Therapeutic Devices	Are integral to the development of diagnostic and therapeutic devices. Biosensors and biochips utilize biomaterials to detect and analyze biological samples for diagnostic purposes	Catheters, prosthetics, and surgical instruments to ensure compatibility and minimize adverse reactions
Wound Healing and Dressings	Are employed in wound healing and dressings. They can create a conducive environment for wound healing by controlling moisture levels, promoting tissue regeneration, and preventing infection	wound healing and dressings
Dental Materials	Are extensively used in dentistry for various applications. Tooth-colored composites and ceramics restore damaged teeth, mimicking natural tooth structure and appearance. Dental adhesives and cements facilitate the bonding of restorative materials to tooth structures	Orthodontic braces and aligners to correct dental misalignments
Surgical Tools and Equipment	Play a role in surgical tools and equipment. Instruments made from biocompatible materials ensure compatibility with the human body during surgical procedures	Implants or sutures that eventually degrade and are absorbed by the body
Research and Development	Are vital in research and development of new medical technologies and treatments. They enable in vitro studies and preclinical testing of medical devices, drug delivery systems, and tissue engineering approaches	New medical technologies and treatments

Table 1.
Biomaterials roles in the human body [21–24].

Overall, biomaterials contribute significantly to modern medicine and healthcare. They enable the repair, replacement, and regeneration of damaged tissues and organs, facilitate drug delivery, improve diagnostic capabilities, and support surgical interventions. By harnessing the unique properties of biomaterials, researchers and medical professionals continue to advance treatments and interventions, ultimately improving patient outcomes and well-being.

The growth and success of the field of biomaterials are evident, as proven by multiple statistics. Researchers are continuously contributing to this field to continue its growth and strengthen its significance for medicine and biology. They address several impediments that appear from patient to patient, contributing significantly to their improvement [8].

2. Classification of materials used for medical applications

The role of biomaterials in the medical field has undergone substantial transformations in response to advances in science and technology. The ever-evolving healthcare landscape and the growing demands of medical practice have been pivotal drivers behind the continuous developments in the field of biomaterials and their diverse applications.

Biomaterials are typically categorized based on their functionality within the human body and their unique material properties [6]. To begin with, one approach to classification is based on their application at various levels of the human body. At the systemic level, biomaterials are used to restore and repair vital systems, such as the skeletal system, where joint replacements and bone plates have become indispensable. On the organ level, we witness remarkable advancements, with artificial heart valves, total valve replacements, and cardiac pacemakers offering life-changing solutions for heart-related ailments. Additionally, the treatment of specific body parts sees biomaterials like artificial hip joints and kidney dialysis machines replacing or aiding damaged or diseased organs, while materials such as screws, sutures, and bone plates play an important role in wound healing.

Another significant classification of biomaterials revolves around their material properties, primarily dividing them into four broad categories: metals, composites, ceramics, and polymers (**Figure 1**). The extensive range of biomaterial options offers practitioners a diverse selection to match specific treatment requirements. For instance, chemically inert metals are chosen for their high electroconductivity and durability, making them suitable for use as electrodes in artificial organs and for long-term restoration of bodily functions. Conversely, biodegradable materials like sutures serve as temporary frameworks, facilitating tissue regeneration in patients who require it.

1. *Metals* are a class of materials characterized by their high electrical conductivity, malleability, ductility, and typically high strength. They consist of metallic elements and often exhibit metallic bonding, where electrons are delocalized and shared among atoms. Metals are commonly used in engineering and biomaterial applications due to their mechanical properties and biocompatibility. Some examples of metals used in biomaterials include titanium, stainless steel, cobalt-chromium alloys, and tantalum. Metals are often utilized for load-bearing applications such as orthopedic implants, dental implants, and cardiovascular stents [25–27].

2. *Composites* are materials composed of two or more distinct components, such as fibers, particles, or flakes, embedded in a matrix material. The combination of

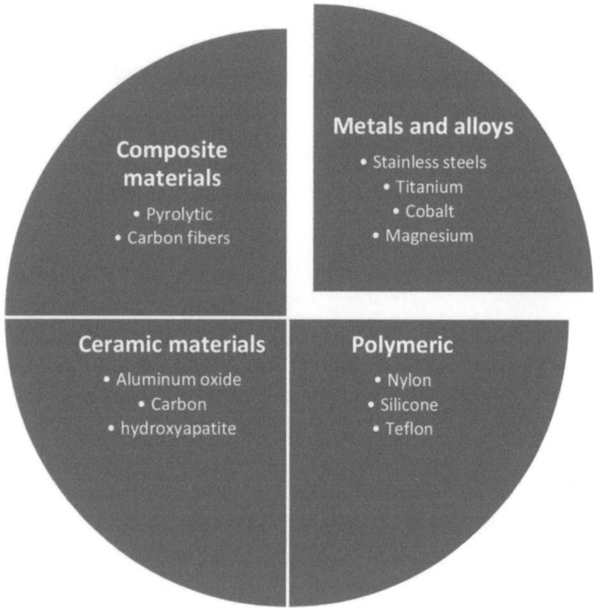

Figure 1.
Classification of biomaterials.

different materials in a composite allows for synergistic properties that are superior to those of the individual components alone. Composites can be engineered to have specific mechanical, electrical, or thermal properties. In biomaterials, composite structures are commonly formed by reinforcing a polymer matrix with fibers or particles made of materials such as carbon fiber, glass fiber, or ceramic particles. The matrix material holds the reinforcement together and transfers loads. Composites find applications in various fields, including aerospace, automotive, and biomedical engineering [28].

3. *Ceramics* are inorganic, non-metallic materials that are typically composed of metallic and non-metallic elements. They are known for their high melting points, hardness, stiffness, and excellent thermal and chemical stability. Ceramics can be crystalline or amorphous in structure. In the context of biomaterials, ceramics such as alumina, zirconia, and hydroxyapatite are used for their biocompatibility, wear resistance, and ability to bond with bone. Ceramic biomaterials are commonly employed in orthopedic implants, dental implants, and coatings for medical devices [29].

4. *Polymers* are large molecules composed of repeating subunits called monomers. They have long chains or networks of interconnected monomers, which give them unique properties. Polymers can be natural or synthetic. Natural polymers, such as collagen and elastin, are found in living organisms. Synthetic polymers, like polyethylene, polyurethane, and silicone, are widely used in biomedical applications. Polymers are known for their versatility, ease of processing, lightweight nature, and tunable properties. They can be tailored to have different mechanical, chemical, and biological characteristics, making them suitable for a

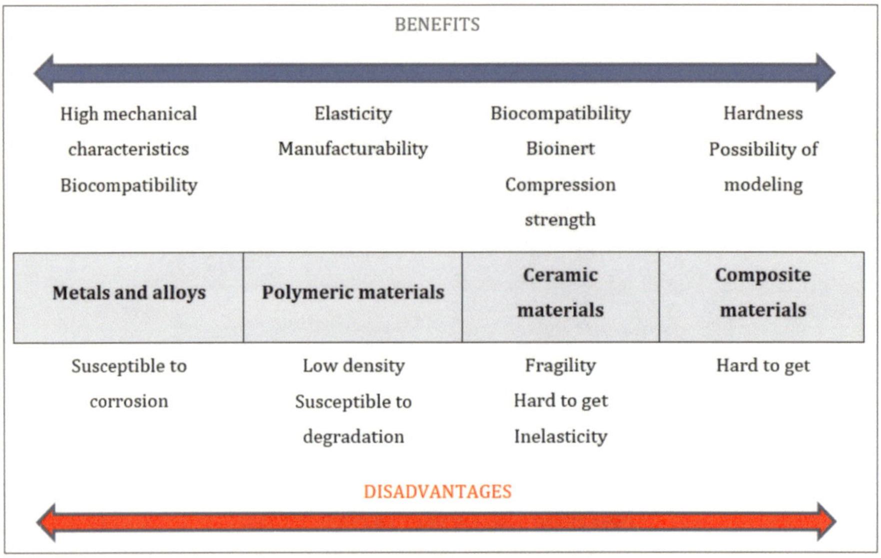

Figure 2.
Few advantages and disadvantages of using different classes of biomaterials.

wide range of biomaterial applications, including tissue engineering scaffolds, drug delivery systems, and medical device coatings [30].

It is important to note that the advantages and disadvantages mentioned above are general and can vary depending on the specific composition, processing techniques, and intended application of the biomaterials. The selection of biomaterials for a particular application should consider the specific requirements, such as mechanical properties, biocompatibility, degradation rate, and the desired interaction with host tissues [31].

The different classes of biomaterials exhibit distinct advantages and disadvantages, which play a defining role in their selection. **Figure 2** provides an overview of the classification of biomaterials in medical applications, organized according to organs, systems, and other body parts. When choosing a biomaterial for a specific application, it is crucial to consider the material's inherent properties, including corrosion resistance, biocompatibility, mechanical and metallurgical properties, as well as its performance during processing and use, cost, and availability. These factors directly influence the suitability of a material for a given application [32–39].

3. Biomaterials advantages and limitations

For medical applications, the design and material choice are vital and are based on the unique requirements of the application. It is important to take into account a few key factors when it comes to metal implants in order to guarantee their security and continued use without rejection. These characteristics include, but are not limited to:

1. *Excellent biocompatibility*: Biocompatibility is a fundamental requirement for any implant material. It refers to the ability of the material to interact with the biological system without causing adverse reactions or toxicity. A metal implant

should be non-toxic and well-tolerated by the body to minimize the risk of inflammation, rejection, or other complications.

2. *High corrosion resistance*: Metal implants are exposed to physiological environments within the body, which can be corrosive. Therefore, it is crucial for the selected metal to possess high corrosion resistance. This ensures that the implant remains structurally stable and maintains its mechanical integrity over time, avoiding the release of potentially harmful metal ions or degradation products.

3. *Adequate mechanical properties*: Metal implants must possess adequate mechanical properties to withstand the physiological loads and stresses they will experience. These properties include strength, toughness, and fatigue resistance. Sufficient mechanical strength is essential to prevent implant failure or deformation under normal physiological conditions.

4. *Wear resistance*: Metal implants, particularly those involved in articulating joints, should exhibit good wear resistance. This helps to minimize the generation of wear particles and the associated inflammatory response, ensuring long-term performance and reducing the risk of complications.

5. *Osseointegration*: In the case of bone prostheses, such as hip or knee implants, osseointegration is a critical characteristic. It refers to the ability of the implant to integrate and form a stable bond with the surrounding bone tissue. This promotes long-term fixation and stability of the implant, allowing for efficient load transfer and improved patient mobility.

In addition to these characteristics, other factors, such as the material's fabrication process, surface properties, and sterilization methods, also play a significant role in the design and selection of metal implants for specific medical applications. Each of these factors should be carefully evaluated and optimized to ensure the safety, efficacy, and long-term success of the implant in the intended patient population [40–45].

By considering these essential characteristics and incorporating them into the design and selection process, engineers and medical professionals can ensure that metal implants meet the specific requirements of the medical application and contribute to improved patient outcomes and quality of life.

Each of the material classes has its own distinct properties and characteristics, making them suitable for specific applications in the field of biomaterials. The choice of material depends on factors such as mechanical requirements, biocompatibility, degradation properties, and the desired interaction with host tissues. **Table 2** highlights some advantages and disadvantages of all classes [3, 17].

There are numerous benefits to using metals and alloys as biomaterials. They are ideal for load-bearing applications such as orthopedic devices and implants because they have outstanding mechanical qualities such as high strength, toughness, and ductility. Many metals and alloys also have a natural resistance to corrosion, which helps them tolerate extreme physiological conditions and ensures their longevity and long-lasting performance in biomedical applications. Certain metals and alloys, including titanium and stainless steel, exhibit strong biocompatibility and are well-tolerated by the body, making it easier for implants used in orthopedics and dentistry

Class	Advantages	Disadvantages
Metals and alloys	• High strength and mechanical properties, suitable for load-bearing applications. • Good corrosion resistance. • Compatible with imaging techniques like X-rays.	• May cause stress shielding, where the implant absorbs stress instead of the surrounding bone, leading to bone loss. • Limited ability to promote tissue regeneration.
Composites	• Tailorable mechanical properties, combining the strengths of different materials. • Can mimic the properties of natural tissues. • Improved biocompatibility and ability to promote tissue regeneration compared to metals.	• Complex fabrication processes. • Potential for delamination or interface failure between the matrix and reinforcement. • Limited availability of biocompatible composite materials.
Ceramics	• Excellent biocompatibility. • High strength and hardness. • Chemical stability and resistance to wear. • Capable of promoting bone regeneration.	• Brittle nature, making them susceptible to fracture. • Poor toughness and low tensile strength. • Difficulty in achieving strong bonding with surrounding tissues.
Polymers	• Versatility and ease of fabrication. • Can be tailored to mimic the properties of natural tissues. • Generally lightweight and flexible. • Some polymers exhibit good biocompatibility and promote tissue integration.	• Lower mechanical strength compared to metals and ceramics. • Limited resistance to wear and degradation. • Potential for leaching of chemicals or degradation byproducts. • May cause inflammation or immune reactions in some cases.

Table 2.
Biomaterials roles in the human body.

to integrate with surrounding tissues and promote osseointegration. Additionally, the properties of metals and alloys can be precisely engineered through careful alterations to their chemical makeup and heat treatment processes, enabling customization to satisfy particular application needs.

Metals and alloys, while offering numerous advantages as biomaterials, also have certain limitations. One limitation is their relatively high density compared to other biomaterials, which can pose challenges in weight-sensitive applications like implants and prosthetics. Additionally, despite their inherent corrosion resistance, metals are still susceptible to wear and corrosion, especially in load-bearing scenarios, necessitating the use of protective coatings or regular monitoring for optimal long-term performance. Another limitation is the potential for allergenic reactions or hypersensitivity to specific metals or alloy components, such as nickel or cobalt, which may restrict their use in certain individuals with sensitivities [46–49].

Composites possess several advantages as biomaterials:

- Tailored Properties: Composites allow for the combination of different materials, such as fibers or particles embedded in a matrix, enabling the attainment of specific mechanical, electrical, or thermal properties. This customization facilitates optimization for diverse applications.

- High Strength-to-Weight Ratio: Composites offer the advantage of high strength combined with low weight. This characteristic is particularly valuable in applications that require lightweight yet robust materials, including aerospace engineering or orthopedic implants.
- Improved Fatigue Resistance: Composites exhibit superior fatigue resistance compared to conventional materials. This attribute renders them well-suited for dynamic load-bearing applications, such as bone fracture fixation or sports equipment.

However, it is important to note that composites also have some limitations, including potential delamination between different material layers, difficulty in recycling due to material heterogeneity, and complexity in fabrication and processing. These limitations need to be carefully considered and addressed in order to fully harness the benefits of composite biomaterials [50–53].

Ceramics are a class of biomaterials that offer numerous advantages for medical applications:

- Biocompatibility: Ceramics such as alumina, zirconia, and bioactive glasses exhibit excellent biocompatibility, meaning they are well-tolerated by the body and do not cause adverse reactions. This makes them suitable for various medical applications.
- High strength and hardness: Ceramics possess exceptional mechanical properties, including high strength and hardness. They can withstand substantial loads and provide structural support in applications such as dental implants and load-bearing joint replacements.
- Wear resistance: Ceramics exhibit low wear rates, making them suitable for articulating surfaces in joints. Their wear resistance helps to minimize the generation of wear debris, reducing the risk of inflammation and implant failure.
- Corrosion resistance: Many ceramics are highly resistant to corrosion, making them suitable for implantation in corrosive physiological environments. They can maintain their structural integrity and prevent the release of potentially harmful ions.
- Tailorable surface properties: Ceramics can be engineered with specific surface characteristics to enhance tissue integration and osseointegration. Surface modifications, such as coatings or roughening, can promote cell adhesion and accelerate the healing process.

Limitations/drawbacks of Ceramics:

- Brittle behavior: Ceramics are inherently brittle materials, meaning they have low fracture toughness and are prone to cracking under tension or impact. This limits their use in applications where high tensile or impact forces are expected.
- Difficulty in processing and shaping: Ceramics often require complex and specialized processing techniques such as sintering, which can be time-consuming and expensive. Additionally, their brittleness makes shaping and machining challenging.

- Lack of resorbability: Unlike certain biomaterials, such as biodegradable polymers, most ceramics are not resorbable by the body. They are intended for long-term use and may require surgical removal if replacement is necessary.
- Poor electrical conductivity: Ceramics have low electrical conductivity, which can be a limitation in certain applications where electrical stimulation or conductivity is required.
- Variability in properties: The properties of ceramics can vary based on factors such as composition, processing, and manufacturing techniques. This variability requires careful quality control and testing to ensure consistent and reliable performance [53, 54].

Polymers offer a wide range of advantages as biomaterials:

- Their versatility allows for a wide range of chemical compositions and the ability to engineer polymers with specific mechanical properties, such as flexibility or stiffness. This makes them highly adaptable for various medical applications, including drug delivery systems, wound dressings, and tissue scaffolds.
- Biocompatibility: Many polymers have excellent biocompatibility, meaning they are well-tolerated by the body and have minimal adverse reactions. They can be designed to closely mimic natural tissues, promoting cell adhesion, proliferation, and tissue regeneration.
- Ease of processing: Polymers are generally easier to process than other biomaterials. They can be molded, extruded, or fabricated into complex shapes using techniques like injection molding or 3D printing. This allows for efficient and cost-effective manufacturing of medical devices and implants.
- Tailorable degradation: Polymers can be designed to degrade at specific rates, allowing for controlled release of drugs or gradual integration with surrounding tissues. This enables precise modulation of the healing process and avoids the need for additional implant removal surgeries.

However, polymers also have certain limitations to consider:

- Mechanical strength: While polymers offer flexibility, they may have lower mechanical strength compared to metals or ceramics. This can limit their use in load-bearing applications or require reinforcement strategies.
- Degradation products: Some polymers may release degradation byproducts during breakdown, which can cause inflammation or tissue response. Careful selection of biocompatible polymers and a thorough understanding of their degradation mechanisms are crucial to minimize these effects [55–58].

Despite these limitations, polymers remain an important class of biomaterials due to their versatility, biocompatibility, ease of processing, and tailorable degradation properties. Ongoing research and development efforts aim to address the limitations and further enhance the performance and applicability of polymer-based biomaterials in various medical fields.

It is important to address these limitations through advanced manufacturing techniques, process optimization, and thorough design analysis to fully exploit the potential of composites in various biomedical applications.

4. Applications of biomaterials in medicine

Biomaterials play a significant and multifaceted role in numerous fields, spanning orthopedics, esthetic surgery, ophthalmology, maxillofacial surgery, cardiology, urology, neurology, and practically all medical specialties encompassing over 400 distinct products. In the realm of medical sciences, biomaterials hold significant importance in the fabrication of dental devices, implants, prostheses, and tissue scaffolds [59–61]. These materials enable advancements in healthcare by providing solutions for various clinical needs, such as restoring mobility, improving esthetics, enhancing vision, repairing facial structures, treating cardiovascular conditions, addressing urological disorders, and facilitating neurological interventions. The broad utilization of biomaterials across diverse medical specialties underscores their indispensable role in enhancing patient care, promoting medical innovation, and improving overall quality of life.

Biomaterials have a vital role in diverse medical applications spanning across various classes:

4.1 Metals and alloys

- *Orthopedics*: The use of titanium alloys in the manufacturing of hip and knee replacements has significantly improved the outcomes of these surgeries by providing durable and biocompatible solutions for joint replacement. A notable example is the development of the Ti-6Al-4 V alloy, widely used in orthopedic implants due to its excellent mechanical properties and good biocompatibility [62, 63].

- *Cardiology*: Cobalt-chromium alloys have been pivotal in the advancement of coronary stents, enhancing the treatment of coronary artery disease. The L605 alloy, for example, is utilized for its superior strength and corrosion resistance, which are critical for maintaining blood vessel patency post-angioplasty [64].

4.2 Composites

- *Dental*: Dental composite materials have revolutionized esthetic dentistry, providing tooth-colored fillings that blend seamlessly with the natural tooth structure. A study by Maran et al. [65] highlights the use of nano-composite resins for fillings, which offer improved esthetics and strength compared to traditional materials.

- *Sports medicine*: Carbon fiber-reinforced polymers are utilized in the fabrication of custom orthotic devices for athletes, combining lightweight properties with high strength. The application of these composites in sports medicine allows for enhanced performance and injury prevention [66].

4.3 Ceramics

- *Dental implants*: Zirconia has become a material of choice for dental implants due to its excellent esthetic properties and biocompatibility. The use of zirconia implants in anterior tooth replacement has been documented for its superior esthetic outcomes and long-term success [53].

- *Bone tissue engineering*: Porous bioceramics, such as hydroxyapatite and tricalcium phosphate, are used in bone grafting procedures to support bone regeneration and healing. These materials provide a scaffold for bone ingrowth, as evidenced by their application in the repair of critical-size bone defects [67].

4.4 Polymers

- *Drug delivery*: Biodegradable polymers like PLGA (poly(lactic-co-glycolic acid)) are used in the development of controlled drug delivery systems, enabling targeted therapy with minimal side effects. The use of PLGA nanoparticles for the delivery of cancer therapeutics has shown promising results in reducing tumor growth [68].

- *Tissue engineering*: Polyethylene glycol (PEG)-based hydrogels are widely used in tissue engineering as scaffolds for cell culture and tissue regeneration. Their application in the development of engineered skin tissue for burn victims has demonstrated significant advances in wound healing and skin restoration [69].

Figure 3 provides a visual representation of various notable applications in medicine where biomaterials are utilized.

Biomaterials include a wide range of materials other than metals because of the many requirements and applications in medicine. Based on their specific qualities and

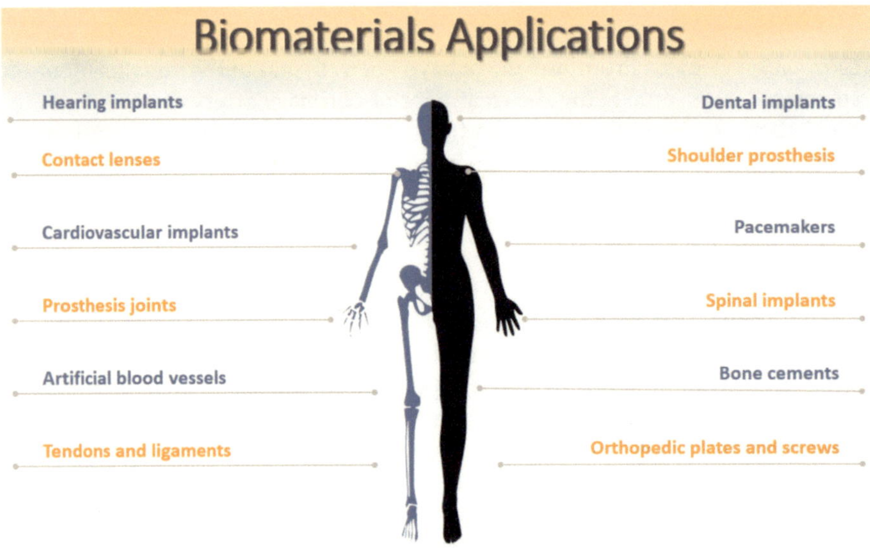

Figure 3.
Various representative applications in medicine.

features, each class of biomaterials has advantages of its own. These biomaterials, which include composites, ceramics, and polymers, were created expressly to address the demands of various medical applications. They offer specialized answers for issues including mechanical strength, biocompatibility, flexibility, and controlled release, advancing medical therapies and improving patient care across a range of medical specializations. As a result, these non-metallic biomaterials continue to be essential for increasing the scope of medical interventions and raising the standard of care in general.

5. Characteristics and tissue interaction factors

The design and selection of biomaterials are contingent upon the specific medical application at hand. In order to excel in the biomedical field over an extended period without eliciting immune rejection (as illustrated in **Figure 4**), biomaterials must possess distinctive characteristics. These characteristics, which contribute to their efficacy, include biocompatibility, appropriate mechanical properties, suitable physical and chemical properties, adequate wear resistance, corrosion resistance, and the ability to promote osseointegration [70]. By fulfilling these criteria, biomaterials can meet the demanding requirements of diverse medical applications, ensuring compatibility with the human body, longevity of performance, and successful integration into the physiological environment.

There are two relative quantitative aspects that distinguish the interactions of biomaterials with the biological environment and create the need for independent study of host and material responses:

1. *Specific requirements* – the biological environment, especially the internal environment of living systems, is very aggressive; it is an environment with

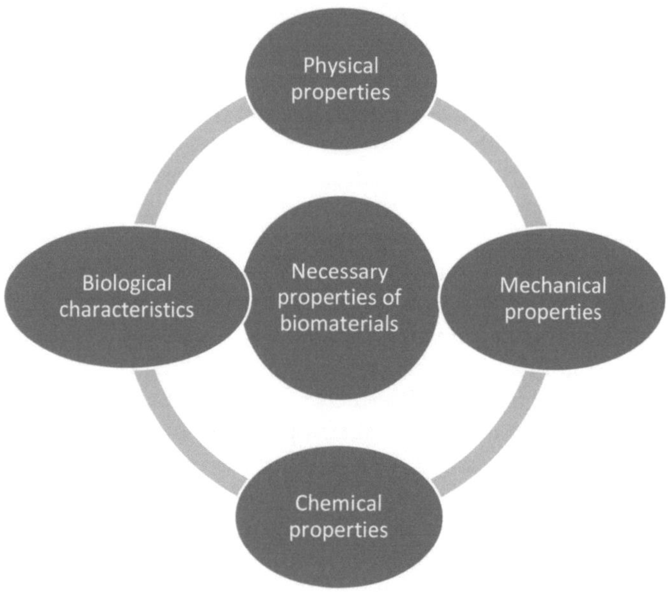

Figure 4.
Schematic demonstration of biomaterial design requirements.

intense and complex chemical activity combined with a wide spectrum, variable depending on some combined mechanical stresses.

2. *Stable conditions* – despite the aggressive aspects, the biological environment presents an extraordinary constant of both the physical conditions and the composition. There are complex control systems that ensure this constant. Therefore, deviations from the stable conditions due to the presence of the material can cause corresponding responses [71].

The aggressive aspects of the biological environment can be understood if we examine the differences between the internal and external conditions of living systems.

Regardless of the views on the development and origin of biological systems, everyone is impressed by their complexity. They perform their functions by accidentally excluding materials that are not needed, or that harm their function in individual processes. Rejection phenomena occur that act to exclude all materials that are toxic or not part of the body. Moreover, the system interacts both locally and regionally or globally. Therefore, a constant aspect of the biological environment is that the introduction of a foreign material will cause a host response, which may have local or systemic consequences [72].

Defining the precise biological environment in which a device or material fulfills a specific function is a challenging task. This challenge stems from the limited understanding of the intricate in vivo conditions and the local variations that can arise during the complex processes involved in maintaining homeostasis, which are essential for sustaining life. The intricate nature of biological systems and the dynamic interplay of various factors make it difficult to comprehensively characterize and predict the exact conditions under which a device or material operates within the body. This highlights the need for ongoing research and a deepening understanding of the complex biological processes to enhance our knowledge and enable more accurate assessments of the performance and functionality of biomedical devices and materials.

Also, there is some ambiguity in defining the region at the interface where the biological environment couples with a material. Implants in isolated body regions can interact with the rest of the system through ion and fluid diffusion, blood circulation, and lymph drainage. Even defining the absolute volume of material communicating with an implant can be difficult. The materials must be tested in vitro before implantation even in animals. It is desirable to try to obtain in the laboratory the operational environment that the material will encounter after implantation [73].

In the case of *in vivo* testing, this is done only under controlled physiological and biophysiological conditions. The biological environment is generally regarded as the sum of the conditions that an implanted material will encounter chronically or acutely, if it is the combination of biological and pericellular conditions. The combination of these extrinsic and intrinsic effects of the environment with the global requirements of the patient during the period proposed for implantation is called the life history of the implant, meaning the totality of the requirements that the biomaterial must meet in order to be successful in the application [74].

The thermal, mechanical, chemical, and surface parameters are sufficient to generally describe the biological environment that the implant encounters. The values differ slightly from patient to patient; the differences that exist have little influence on the response of the host and the material. It is a shame that the technology for determining implant functionality and biomaterial-biological environment interactions is poorly developed compared to that available to biological scientists who study organs in situ.

Within a specific application, the selection of materials and the design of the elements that incorporate them are called "appropriate expectations." This term does not take into account the changes that occur in the patient's life after implantation, but it does guide the selection of technologies before implantation. Better said, we try to design the most durable biomaterials and the best surfaces to meet the requirements.

When performing the tests necessary to assess the interactions at the biomaterial-tissue interface, the objective and subjective factors that can influence the response of the tissue, but also that of the biomaterial, are taken into account in order to be able to make a correct interpretation of the results, depending on the material factors and specifically, those related to the surface [75].

In general, there are two intermediate processes common to all implantation applications. First, the implant can be contaminated accidentally or as a result of manufacturing or handling processes during storage or insertion. It is usually assumed that the surface of the implant is pure and clean. The truth can be totally different. Organic elements from manufacturing or improper handling may persist. Oxidation or other harmful elements can occur during the preoperative stages, materials can be lifted from the packaging used to store them, and pathogens can be transferred from surgical instruments.

For this reason, experimental studies on biomaterial-tissue interaction should include surface characteristics of actual implant samples, selected from a batch manufactured for a particular study, under conditions prior to surgical insertion [76].

Second, all implants must be sterilized before use. Some of them may be supplied by the manufacturer in sterile double-wrap packages, while others must be sterilized in a laboratory or hospital before use. Skipping the sterilization process can affect both host and material responses. Sterilization of an implant may render it sterile but not risk-free, thus altering the host's response. Therefore, in examining the response of the material or the host to the implant, it is necessary to pay more attention to the conditions of surface preparation.

The outcome of an implant replacement is heavily influenced by the interaction between the synthetic material and the surrounding tissue, leading to a diverse range of effects. Implants that come into contact with blood typically require a hemocompatible behavior characterized by minimal interaction to ensure compatibility. In contrast, osseointegrated implants necessitate a strong interaction to achieve high adhesion forces. The process of osseointegration can be influenced by multiple factors, including the surface structure, topography, and composition of the implant material. These aspects play a critical role in facilitating a successful integration with the bone tissue, highlighting the significance of carefully designing implant surfaces to optimize the desired level of interaction and promote favorable outcomes [74].

Many significant factors that individually play a significant role in the effectiveness of implantation influence the direct interaction between tissue and biomaterials. The macrostructure and microstructure of the implant, the surgical implantation technique, the initial tissue-implant contact, the loading conditions on the implant, and the implantation support are some of these aspects. Also included are the biocompatibility of the chosen material. A major obstacle to the placement and operation of metal implants is achieving a sustainable anchoring of the implant in the tissue.

One approach to address tissue anchoring is the use of structured surfaces that promote cell growth, such as porous surfaces. Implants with sandblasted or spherical particle coatings facilitate tissue contact and growth within the interstices of the implant. Another method to enhance surface structure involves creating controlled microstructures with a roughness on the order of a few micrometers. Studies have shown that the superficial layer structure of a metal implant should allow for secondary fixation through the penetration of bone trabeculae into the microcavities of the surface. This surface topography resembles resorbed bone surfaces, which have been utilized as anchor points for newly formed bone. Hence, implant surfaces mimicking the bone structure after resorption are expected to achieve better long-term fixation and stability.

The principle of direct tissue-implant contact requires rigid mechanical fixation, as a soft tissue layer can induce micromovements at the interface. Micromovements can lead to undesirable reactions such as the destruction of the implant's oxide layer, corrosion, and implant rejection. Rough implants with larger surface areas in contact with tissue are also more susceptible to corrosion processes. Additionally, rigidly fixed metal implants with specific geometries can cause shielding and subsequent bone resorption. These issues highlight the importance of surface preparation, including implant geometry and the arrangement and amplitude of surface elevations and depressions [76].

The surface structure of an implant significantly influences both its fixation and the adhesion force to the surrounding tissue. A soft implant surface with a smaller contact area exhibits lower adhesion force compared to a structured surface. Studies investigating the importance of roughness have demonstrated that increasing roughness enhances adhesion force. Moreover, resistance to breakage increases with greater contact area achieved by introducing holes in flattened cylinders. Adhesion force is also influenced by the duration of implantation, as bone requires time to fill the free space between the implant and surface cavities, leading to mechanical relaxation of the implant.

Beyond the beneficial effects on implant fixation, surface structuring provides advantages in terms of stimulating bone formation. Compressive stress on growing bone generates calcium production, promoting bone growth. This phenomenon becomes more pronounced as charge transfer improves through enhanced surface topography [73].

The biological environment within the human body is chemically, mechanically, and electrically active. The interface between biomaterials and tissue serves as a site for numerous biochemical and biodynamic processes and reactions. Oxygen diffuses from the oxidized surface into the base metal, while metal ions can diffuse onto the surface. Interactions between biological molecules and the implant surface can induce transient or permanent changes in their conformation, resulting in functional alterations.

Understanding and manipulating these complex interactions within the biological environment is critical for optimizing the design and performance of biomaterials in medical applications.

6. Future trends in biomaterials applications

The demand for novel solutions in healthcare and medicine is propelling the rapid advancement of the biomaterials industry. Biomaterials are anticipated to display sophisticated functions in the upcoming years beyond their current uses. These materials will be created with characteristics including self-healing, stimulus responsiveness, and controlled medication release, allowing for customized and focused therapeutic results. The creation of bioactive and bioresorbable materials will also alter the industry since they work with the body's natural mechanisms to encourage tissue regeneration, degrade over time, or be replaced by fresh tissue.

The emergence of technologies like 3D printing and additive manufacturing will revolutionize the production of biomaterials. These techniques enable precise control over material composition, structure, and geometry, allowing for patient-specific implants, tissue scaffolds, and drug delivery systems. Nanotechnology will also play a significant role, offering unique properties through nanostructured materials such as increased surface area, enhanced mechanical strength, and improved biocompatibility [61].

Biomimetic materials, inspired by nature, will gain prominence in future biomaterials applications. By mimicking the structure and function of natural tissues and organs, these materials enhance biocompatibility and improve integration with the host environment. Furthermore, the combination of biomaterials with other therapeutic approaches such as gene therapy, stem cell therapy, and immunotherapy will lead to innovative treatment strategies and tissue regeneration techniques.

Sustainability and environmental impact will also be important considerations in the future of biomaterials. There will be a shift toward developing biodegradable and environmentally sustainable materials to reduce the long-term ecological footprint of medical devices and promote the use of eco-friendly alternatives.

Additionally, the integration of smart features and sensors into biomaterials will enable real-time monitoring and response to physiological changes. This opens up opportunities for early disease detection, personalized diagnostics, and continuous health monitoring, revolutionizing patient care and management.

As we delve into the exciting realm of biomaterials and their ever-expanding applications, it is essential to address a multitude of evolving factors that are shaping the future of this field. From the innovative potential of nanotechnology in drug delivery to the transformative influence of surface engineering, additive manufacturing, and the integration of Industry 4.0/5.0 and Society 5.0, the landscape of biomaterials is undergoing a profound metamorphosis. Moreover, we explore the pivotal role of digitization, personalization, and the ecological considerations that are becoming increasingly indispensable in the development of medical devices and implants:

- *Nanotechnology's role in drug delivery*: In the dynamic landscape of biomaterials, nanotechnology has emerged as a game-changer, particularly in the realm of drug delivery systems. Nanoparticles and nanocarriers hold the potential to revolutionize how medicines are administered, enhancing precision and efficacy.

- *Surface engineering and additive manufacturing*: Innovations in surface engineering and additive manufacturing techniques have brought exciting possibilities to biomaterials. These advancements allow for the fine-tuning of material properties at the surface level and the creation of intricate structures, paving the way for more customized medical devices and implants.

- *Integration of Industry 4.0/5.0 and Society 5.0*: An integral part of envisioning the future of biomaterials involves their synergy with the concepts of Industry 4.0 and 5.0, as well as Society 5.0. These paradigms usher in a new era of interconnectedness and intelligent manufacturing, where biomaterials play a central role in the development of smart medical devices and treatments.

- *Digital transformation and personalization*: As we move forward, the digitization and personalization of medical devices, including biomaterial-based implants, are becoming indispensable. Tailoring medical solutions to individual patients' needs not only improves treatment outcomes but also minimizes risks and enhances patient satisfaction.

- *Environmental considerations*: While the focus on patient safety remains paramount, the ecological footprint of biomaterial production should not be overlooked. Inadequate material choices can harm the environment on a larger scale, affecting countless lives. Therefore, sustainability and adherence to ecological requirements are increasingly vital aspects of biomaterial development.

Together, these trends herald a new era in biomaterials science, with far-reaching implications for healthcare and environmental sustainability.

In conclusion, the future of biomaterials applications is filled with exciting possibilities. Advanced functionalities, bioactive materials, 3D printing, nanotechnology, biomimetics, combination therapies, sustainable materials, and smart integration are key trends that will shape the field. These advancements hold great promise for revolutionizing healthcare, enabling personalized treatments, improved patient outcomes, and a brighter future in medical innovation.

7. Conclusion

The chapter on trends in biomaterials applications has shed light on the remarkable advancements and challenges within the field. Biomaterials have proven to be indispensable in various medical applications, offering numerous advantages while also presenting certain limitations. Understanding these trends, advantages, and limitations is significant for researchers, scientists, and healthcare professionals to navigate the ever-evolving landscape of biomaterials.

Furthermore, it is imperative to underscore the critical role of considering allergic reactions in biomedical applications. Careful selection of biomaterials for medical devices should not only account for their mechanical properties but also factor in the potential for allergic responses. This involves a comprehensive understanding of the social, health, and regulatory implications associated with specific materials, such as nickel-containing alloys. In fact, in response to health concerns related to allergic reactions, certain regions, notably the European Union, have enacted stringent regulations leading to the removal of particular materials from biomedical applications.

The advantages of biomaterials, such as metals and alloys, composites, ceramics, and polymers, have been highlighted throughout the chapter. These materials offer unique properties that make them suitable for specific applications. Their mechanical strength, corrosion resistance, biocompatibility, and tailorable properties have played a vital role in the success of implantable devices, orthopedic applications, and tissue engineering.

However, it is equally important to recognize the limitations associated with biomaterials. Factors such as density, wear and corrosion, allergenic reactions, manufacturing complexity, and anisotropy must be considered when designing and selecting biomaterials for medical applications. Addressing these limitations requires continuous research, innovation, and collaboration across disciplines.

The future of biomaterials applications holds tremendous promise. Advancements in biomaterials will continue to drive the development of innovative medical devices, regenerative therapies, and personalized medicine. The integration of advanced functionalities, such as self-healing, stimuli-responsiveness, and controlled drug release, will revolutionize treatment approaches and improve patient outcomes.

Technological advancements, including 3D printing, nanotechnology, and smart materials, will reshape the manufacturing processes and capabilities of biomaterials. These technologies enable the production of patient-specific implants, nanostructured materials, and real-time monitoring systems, leading to personalized diagnostics, tailored therapies, and enhanced healthcare delivery.

Sustainability and environmental considerations are increasingly important in biomaterials research. The development of biodegradable and eco-friendly materials will contribute to reducing the ecological impact of medical devices and aligning healthcare practices with environmental stewardship.

We can conclude that biomaterials are materials engineered to interact with biological systems for medical purposes. These uses highlight the important role that biomaterials play in advancing medical research, better patient outcomes, and improving the quality of life for people with a range of medical illnesses. Future research promises even more advancements as it explores novel biomaterials and inventive medical applications.

In conclusion, understanding the trends, advantages, and limitations of biomaterials applications is essential for advancing the field and improving patient care. By leveraging the strengths of biomaterials while addressing their limitations, researchers and healthcare professionals can harness the full potential of these materials to shape the future of medicine, enabling breakthroughs in diagnostics, treatments, and patient well-being. Continued collaboration, research, and innovation will drive the evolution of biomaterials and pave the way for a new era in healthcare.

Conflict of interest

The authors declare no conflict of interest.

Author details

Mihaela Claudia Spataru[1], Madalina Simona Baltatu[2], Andrei Victor Sandu[2,3]
and Petrica Vizureanu[2,4]*

1 Faculty of Veterinary Medicine, "Ion Ionescu de la Brad" University of Life Sciences, Iasi, Romania

2 Faculty of Materials Science and Engineering, Gheorghe Asachi Technical University of lasi, lasi, Romania

3 Academy of Romanian Scientists, Bucharest, Romania

4 Technical Sciences Academy of Romania, Bucharest, Romania

*Address all correspondence to: peviz2002@yahoo.com

References

[1] Wang M, Guo L, Sun H. Manufacture of biomaterials. In: Narayan R, editor. Encyclopedia of Biomedical Engineering. The Netherlands: Elsevier; 2019. pp. 116-134

[2] Geetha M, Singh AK, Asokamani R, Gogia AK. Ti based biomaterials, the ultimate choice for orthopaedic implants – A review. Progress in Materials Science. 2009;**54**:397-425

[3] Chen Q, Thouas GA. Metallic implant biomaterials. Materials Science & Engineering R: Reports. 2015;**87**:1-57

[4] Antoniac I, Miculescu M, Mănescu (Păltânea) V, Stere A, Quan PH, Păltânea G, et al. Magnesium-based alloys used in Orthopedic surgery. Materials. 2022;**15**:1148

[5] Niinomi M. Mechanical properties of biomedical titanium alloys. Materials Science and Engineering A. 1998;**243**: 231-236

[6] Ratner BD, Bryant SJ. Biomaterials: Where we have been and where we are going. Annual Review of Biomedical Engineering. 2004;**6**:41-75

[7] Ratner BD, Zhang G. A history of biomaterials. In: Biomaterials Science. Amsterdam, Netherlands: Academic Press; 2020. pp. 21-34

[8] Shahani S. Advanced drug delivery systems: New developments, new technologies report No. PHM006F. Business Communications Company. 2006

[9] Dondossola E, Holzapfel B, Alexander S, Filippini S, Hutmacher D, Friedl P. Examination of the foreign body response to biomaterials by nonlinear intravital microscopy. Nature Biomedical Engineering. 2017;**1**:0007. DOI: 10.1038/s41551-016-0007

[10] Hildebrand HF. Biomaterials–A history of 7000 years. BioNanoMaterials. 2013;**14**:119-133

[11] Crubézy E, Murail P, Girard L, Bernadou JP. False teeth of the Roman world. Nature Cell Biology. 1998; **391**:29

[12] Huang J, Best SM. Ceramic biomaterials. In: Tissue Engineering Using Ceramics and Polymers. Netherlands: Woodhead Publishing; 2007. pp. 3-31

[13] Ramakrishna S, Ramalingam M, Kumar TS, Soboyejo WO. Biomaterials: A Nano Approach. Boca Raton, Florida, USA: CRC Press; 2019

[14] Prasad K, Bazaka O, Chua M, Rochford M, Fedrick L, Spoor J, et al. Metallic Biomaterials: Current Challenges and Opportunities. Materials (Basel). 31 Jul 2017;**10**(8):884. DOI: 10.3390/ma10080884. PMID: 28773240; PMCID: PMC5578250

[15] Peppas NA, Khademhosseini A. Make better, safer biomaterials. Nature. 2016;**540**:335

[16] Baltatu MS, Spataru MC, Verestiuc L, Balan V, Solcan C, Sandu AV, et al. Design, synthesis, and preliminary evaluation for Ti-Mo-Zr-Ta-Si alloys for potential implant applications. Materials. 2021;**14**(22):6806

[17] Istrate B, Munteanu C, Cimpoesu R, Cimpoesu N, Popescu OD, Vlad MD. Microstructural, electrochemical and In vitro analysis of Mg-0.5Ca-xGd

biodegradable alloys. Applied Sciences. 2021;**11**:981

[18] Baltatu MS, Vizureanu P, Goanţă V, Tugui CA, Voiculescu I. Mechanical tests for Ti-based alloys as new medical materials. IOP Conference Series: Materials Science and Engineering. 2019; **572**:012029

[19] Baltatu MS, Sandu AV, Nabialek M, Vizureanu P, Ciobanu G. Biomimetic deposition of hydroxyapatite layer on titanium alloys. Micromachines. 2021;**12**: 1447

[20] Wu B, Jin L, Ding K, Zhou Y, Yang L, Lei Y, et al. Extracellular matrix coating improves the biocompatibility of polymeric heart valves. Journal of Materials Chemistry B. 2020;**8**:10616-10629

[21] Langer R, Tirrell DA. Designing materials for biology and medicine. Nature. 2004;**428**:487-492

[22] Savin A, Vizureanu P, Prevorovsky Z, Chlada M, Krofta J, Baltatu MS, et al. Noninvasive evaluation of special alloys for prostheses using complementary methods. IOP Conference Series: Materials Science and Engineering. 2018; **374**:012030

[23] Liu Z, Liu X, Ramakrishna S. Surface engineering of biomaterials in orthopedic and dental implants: Strategies to improve osteointegration, bacteriostatic and bactericidal activities. Biotechnology Journal. 2021;**16**:2000116

[24] Todros S, Todesco M, Bagno A. Biomaterials and their biomedical applications: From replacement to regeneration. PRO. 2021;**9**:1949. DOI: 10.3390/pr9111949

[25] Istrate B, Munteanu C, Antoniac I-V, Lupescu S-C. Current research studies of Mg–Ca–Zn biodegradable alloys used as Orthopedic implants—Review. Crystals. 2022;**12**:1468

[26] Bita AI, Antoniac A, Cotrut C, Vasile E, Ciuca I, Niculescu M, et al. In vitro degradation and corrosion evaluation of Mg-Ca alloys for biomedical applications. Journal of Optoelectronics and Advanced Materials. 2016;**18**(3–4):394-398

[27] Antoniac I, Miculescu F, Cotrut C, Ficai A, Rau JV, Grosu E, et al. Controlling the degradation rate of biodegradable Mg–Zn-Mn alloys for Orthopedic applications by electrophoretic deposition of hydroxyapatite coating. Materials. 2020; **13**(1):263

[28] Istratov VV, Vasnev VA, Markova GD. Biodegradable and biocompatible Silatrane polymers. Molecules. 2021;**26** (7):1893

[29] Bronzino JD, Peterson DR, editors. The Biomedical Engineering Handbook. 4th ed. Boca Raton, Florida: CRC Press; 2015

[30] Cui W, Santos HA, Zhang B, Zhang YS. Functional biomaterials. APL Bioengineering. 2022;**6**(1):010401

[31] Vallet-Regi M. Evolution of biomaterials. Frontiers in Materials. 2022;**9**:864016

[32] Ramakrishna S, Ramalingam M, Sampath Kumar TS, Soboyejo WO. Biomaterials: A Nano Approach. 1st ed. Boca Raton, Florida: CRC Press; 2010

[33] Virtanen S. Corrosion of biomedical implant materials. Corrosion Reviews. 2008;**26**:147-171

[34] Kokubo T, Yamaguchi S. Bioactive metals prepared by surface modification: Preparation and properties. In: Eliaz N,

editor. Applications of Electrochemistry in Biology and Medicine I. New York City: Springer Science+Business Media; 2011. pp. 377-421

[35] Wang LQ, Liu CZ, Xie LC. Metallic biomaterials for medical applications. Frontiers in Materials. 2021;**8**: 795642

[36] Dondossola E, Holzapfel B, Alexander S, Filippini S, Hutmacher D, Friedl P. Examination of the foreign body response to biomaterials by nonlinear intravital microscopy. Nat Biomed Eng 2017;**1**:0007. DOI: 10.1038/s41551-016-0007

[37] Baltatu I, Sandu AV, Vlad MD, Spataru MC, Vizureanu P, Baltatu MS. Mechanical characterization and In vitro assay of biocompatible titanium alloys. Micromachines. 2022;**13**(3):430

[38] Ciolac S, Vasilescu E, Drob P, Popa MV, Anghel M. Long-term in vitro study of titanium and some titanium alloys used in surgical implants. Revue Roumaine de Chimie. 2000;**51**(1–2):36-41

[39] Chelariu R, Bujoreanu G, Roman C. Materiale metalice biocompatibile cu baza titan. Politehnium. 2006

[40] Bobyn JD, Stackpool GJ, Hacking SA, et al. Characteristics of bone ingrowth and interface mechanics of a new porous tantalum biomaterial. Journal of Bone and Joint Surgery – British Volume. 1999;**81**(5): 907-914

[41] Ou P, Liu J, Hao C, He R, Chang L, Ruan J. Cytocompatibility, stability and osteogenic activity of powder metallurgy Ta-xZr alloys as dental implant materials. Journal of Biomaterials Applications. 2021;**35**(7):790-798. DOI: 10.1177/0885328220948033

[42] Manivasagam G, Dhinasekaran D, Rajamanickam A. Biomedical implants: Corrosion and its prevention—A review. Recent Patents on Corrosion Science. 2010;**2**(1):40-54

[43] Hoemann CD, El-Gabalawy H, McKee MD. In vitro osteogenesis assays: Influence of the primary cell source on alkaline phosphatase activity and mineralization. Pathologie et Biologie. 2009;**57**:318-323

[44] Wang Q, Zhang H, Li Q, et al. Biocompatibility and osteogenic properties of porous tantalum. Experimental and Therapeutic Medicine. 2015;**9**:780-786

[45] Verma RP. Titanium-based biomaterial for bone implants: A mini review. Materials Today Proceedings. 2020;**26**:3148-3151

[46] Baltatu MS, Vizureanu P, Balan T, Lohan NM, Tugui CA. Preliminary tests for Ti-Mo-Zr-Ta alloys as potential biomaterials. IOP Conference Series: Materials Science and Engineering. 2018; **374**:012023

[47] Weng W, Biesiekierski A, Li Y, Wen C. Effects of selected metallic and interstitial elements on the microstructure and mechanical properties of beta titanium alloys for orthopedic applications. Materialia. 2019;**6**:100323

[48] Ashtiani RE, Alam M, Tavakolizadeh S, Abbasi K. The role of biomaterials and biocompatible materials in implant-supported dental prosthesis. Evidence-based Complementary and Alternative Medicine. 2021;**2021**:3349433

[49] Li DX, Uy B, Wang J, Song YC. Assessment of titanium alloy bolts for structural applications. Steel and

Composite Structures. 2022;**42**(4): 553-568

[50] Burg KJL, Porter S, Kellam JF. Biomaterial developments for bone tissue engineering. Biomaterials. 2000; **21**:2347-2359

[51] Thomas MB, Metoki N, Geuli O, Sharabani-Yosef O, Zada T, Reches M, et al. Quickly manufactured, drug eluting, calcium phosphate composite coating. ChemistrySelect. 2017;**2**:753-758

[52] Al-Salloum YA, Almusallam TH. Rehabilitation of the infrastructure using composite materials: Overview and applications. Journal of King Saud University – Engineering Sciences. 2003; **16**:1-20

[53] Bona AD, Pecho OE, Alessandretti R. Zirconia as a dental biomaterial. Maternité. 2015;**8**(8):4978-4991

[54] Huang Z, Wang Z, Li C, Yin K, Hao D, Lan J. Application of plasma sprayed zirconia coating in dental implant: Study in implant. The Journal of Oral Implantology. 2018;**44**:264-270

[55] Camilo CC, Silveira CA, Faeda RS, Almeida Rollo JM, Purquerio BM, Fortulan CA. Bone response to porous alumina implants coated with bioactive materials, observed using different characterization techniques. Journal of Applied Biomaterials & Functional Materials. 2017;**15**(3):223-235

[56] Chatterjee S, Hui PC. Review of applications and future prospects of stimuli-responsive hydrogel based on Thermo-responsive biopolymers in drug delivery systems. Polymers. 2021;**13**: 2086

[57] Dhivya S, Padma VV, Santhini E. Wound dressings—A review. Biomedicine. 2015;**5**:1-5

[58] Gritsch L, Maqbool M, Mouriño V, Ciraldo FE, Cresswell M, Jackson PR, et al. Chitosan/hydroxyapatite composite bone tissue engineering scaffolds with dual and decoupled therapeutic ion delivery: Copper and strontium. Journal of Materials Chemistry B. 2019;**7**: 6109-6124

[59] Sidambe AT. Biocompatibility of advanced manufactured titanium implants—A review. Materials. 2014;**7**: 8168-8188

[60] Bastola AK, Paudel M, Li L, et al. Recent progress of magnetorheological elastomers: A review. Smart Materials and Structures. 2020;**29**(12):123002

[61] Bhattacharyya A, Janarthanan G, Noh I. Nanobiomaterials for designing functional bioinks towards complex tissue and organ regeneration in 3D bioprinting. Additive Manufacturing. 2021;**37**:101639

[62] Ackun-Farmmer MA, Overby CT, Haws BE, et al. Biomaterials for orthopedic diagnostics and theranostics. Current Opinion in Biomedical Engineering. 2021;**19**:100308

[63] Marsh M, Newman S. Trends and developments in hip and knee arthroplasty technology. Journal of Rehabilitation and Assistive Technologies Engineering. 2021;**8**: 2055668320952043. DOI: 10.1177/2055668320952043

[64] Lushchik PE, Botirov MT, Rafalski IV, Mamajonov MM, Niss VS, Normatova SA. Co-Cr alloys for biocompatible medical products, E3S web of conferences, 050 (2023). IPFA. 2023;**452**:15. DOI: 10.1051/e3sconf/202345205015

[65] Maran BM, Larocca J, de Geus M, Gutiérrez F, Heintze S, Tardem C, et al.

Nanofilled/nanohybrid and hybrid resin-based composite in patients with direct restorations in posterior teeth: A systematic review and meta-analysis. Journal of Dentistry. 2020;**99**:103407. DOI: 10.1016/j.jdent.2020.103407

[66] Zhang Z. The application and influence of polymer composite materials in competitive sports. Applied and Computational Engineering. 2023; **25**:1-8:8265188686

[67] Ginebra MP, Espanol M, Maazouz Y, Bergez V, Pastorino D. Bioceramics and bone healing. EFORT Open Reviews. 2018;**3**(5):173-183. DOI: 10.1302/2058-5241.3.170056

[68] Vroman I, Tighzert L. Biodegradable Polymers. Materials. 2009;**2**:307-344. DOI: 10.3390/ma2020307

[69] Li H, Liu C, Qi X, Cuifen L, Yang G, Wang F, et al. Bioengineered three-dimensional scaffolds to elucidate the effects of material biodegradability on cell behavior using POSS-PEG hybrid hydrogels. Polymer Degradation and Stability. 2019;**164**:118-126. DOI: 10.1016/j.polymdegradstab.2019.04.008

[70] Janarthanan G, Noh I. Recent trends in metal ion-based hydrogel biomaterials for tissue engineering and other biomedical applications. Journal of Materials Science and Technology. 2021; **63**:35-53

[71] Srivastav A. Chapter 7. An overview of metallic biomaterials for bone support and replacement. Biomedical Engineering, Trends in Materials Science. London: IntechOpen; 2011. pp. 153-168; DOI: 10.5772/13488

[72] Spataru M-C, Cojocaru FD, Sandu AV, Solcan C, Duceac IA, Baltatu MS, et al. Assessment of the effects of Si addition to a new TiMoZrTa system. Materials. 2021;**14**:7610

[73] Liu X, Song X, Zhang P, et al. Effects of nano tantalum implants on inducing osteoblast proliferation and differentiation. Experimental and Therapeutic Medicine. 2016;**12**: 3541-3544

[74] KFim H, Kumbar SG, Nukavarapu SP. Biomaterial-directed cell behavior for tissue engineering. Current Opinion in Biomedical Engineering. 2021;**17**: 100260. DOI: 10.1016/j.cobme.2020.100260. Epub 2020 Dec 25

[75] Morais JM, Papadimitrakopoulos F, Burgess DJ. Biomaterials/tissue interactions: Possible solutions to overcome foreign body response. The AAPS Journal. 2010;**12**(2):188-196. DOI: 10.1208/s12248-010-9175-3. Epub 2010 Feb 9

[76] Londono R, Badylak SF. Chapter 1 – Factors which affect the host response to biomaterials. In: Badylak SF, editor. Host Response to Biomaterials. United States: Academic Press; 2015. pp. 1-12. ISBN 9780128001967. DOI: 10.1016/B978-0-12-800196-7.00001-3

Chapter 2

Mg-Li-Based Alloys as Implant Materials

Chiamaka Okafor and Norman Munroe

Abstract

This chapter is aimed at discussing the prospect of using novel magnesium-lithium-based alloys for temporary implantation. It discusses the challenges of implant materials and focuses on the design, characterization, and assessment of Mg-Li-Zn-Ca alloys. Biodegradable magnesium alloys have recently been the material of choice for the manufacture of implantable medical devices because they proffer efficacious solutions to temporary implantation. Magnesium-lithium-based alloys are a unique system of alloys that offer enhanced ductility and uniform degradation. The increase of lithium in the quaternary Mg-Li-Zn-Ca system resulted in phase transformation of the hcp crystal structure of magnesium to bcc, thus improving ductility. Lithium promoted the formation of a solid solution and a compact surface oxide that decreased corrosion kinetics in biological media. The alloys exhibited good biocompatibility, as evidenced by cell viability and metabolic activity when exposed to solutions retrieved from immersion tests. Furthermore, the improvement in mechanical properties and degradation properties of these alloys relative to other magnesium-based alloys provide an opportunity for wider adoption in the biomedical field.

Keywords: magnesium-lithium, biodegradable alloys, metallic implants, phase transformation, corrosion, biocompatibility

1. Introduction

In the last two decades, there has been a paradigm shift aimed at developing biomaterials for temporary implant applications such as screws and vascular stents. This is because it is not beneficial for metallic materials that have finished serving their purpose to remain in the body permanently. Complications associated with the use of permanent implants for temporary treatments include extractive surgeries, thrombosis, extended use of antiplatelet drugs, and blood thinners. In addition, there are pediatric cases where children are deemed unfit for permanent implant placement. Bioresorbable alloys are required to manage orthopedic, cardiovascular, and neural diseases.

Historically, metals and other materials have been used to repair the human body, dating back several millennia [1]. Until the mid-nineteenth century, copper and bronze were suitable implantation materials, but poisoning from copper ion leaching was a concern [2]. In 1880, Gluck, used ivory prosthesis as implants in the body, and in 1902, gold was used as the interphase between the articular heads of the implant.

Aspect	Description
Resorption	Mechanical integrity 3 to 6 months Full dissolution within 1 to 2 years
Biocompatibility	Non-toxic, no inflammatory tissue response No harmful release and/or residue of particles
Mechanical Properties	Tensile yield stress TYS > 200 MPa Ultimate strength UTS > 300 MPa Tensile elongation >15–18%
Microstructure	Maximum grain size of 10–12.5 μm
Hydrogen Evolution	Evolution <10 μL H^2 cm^{-2} day^{-1}
Corrosion Rate	Corrosion rate < 0.2 mm/year

Table 1.
Design parameter for biodegradable magnesium stent [5–7].

This experiment proved to be successful, which led to further studies on chemically inert and stable materials [3].

Biodegradable materials dissolve within the human body after serving therapeutic functions, and the healing process is complete. A bioresorbable vascular stent, for instance, should be able to provide the required mechanical strength for restructuring a diseased artery over a specified period and subsequently be gradually resorbed by the body after its function is completed. Bioresorbable materials should be biocompatible, functional, durable, and safe before being considered for implantation. These characteristics determine the type of material that should be used for specific applications. For example, metallic materials, when compared to polymeric materials, have better desirable mechanical properties and are radiopaque [4], thus making imaging easier. **Table 1** highlights the essential properties of magnesium alloys used for the manufacture of stents.

Magnesium is a good fit for biological implants because the human body can innocuously process a relatively high level of magnesium content. Magnesium serves multiple biological functions within the body, such as regulating muscles, heart rhythm, cholesterol production, and blood pressure. Moreover, more than 300 enzyme processes within the body require magnesium [8], and it has a recommended daily average intake of 310–420 mg [9] compared to zinc (8–40 mg/day) and iron (5–27 mg/day) [10]. However, the greatest challenge facing the adoption of magnesium-based alloy in the medical industry is the need for controlled and uniform degradation, as well as sustained mechanical integrity [11]. The degradation issues arise from the inherent vigorous electrochemical reactivity of Mg alloys. Magnesium is found to react spontaneously in aqueous solutions because of the ease of transfer of its electrons. Research efforts have considered the use of various alloying elements, heat treatments, and metallurgical processing techniques, such as extrusion, to alter their microstructure, which ultimately impacts degradation and mechanical properties.

The global bioimplant market size is currently estimated at over $260 billion, with increasing demand for minimally invasive surgeries, chronic disorders, bone degeneration, and a rising aging population as driving forces [12–14]. Orthopedic and cardiovascular implants account for ~50% of the market share by type, whereas metallic implants have the largest share by materials, as shown in **Figure 1** [13, 15]. The regional outlook puts North America ahead of Europe and Asia as having the highest market share, with Asia having the fastest-growing market.

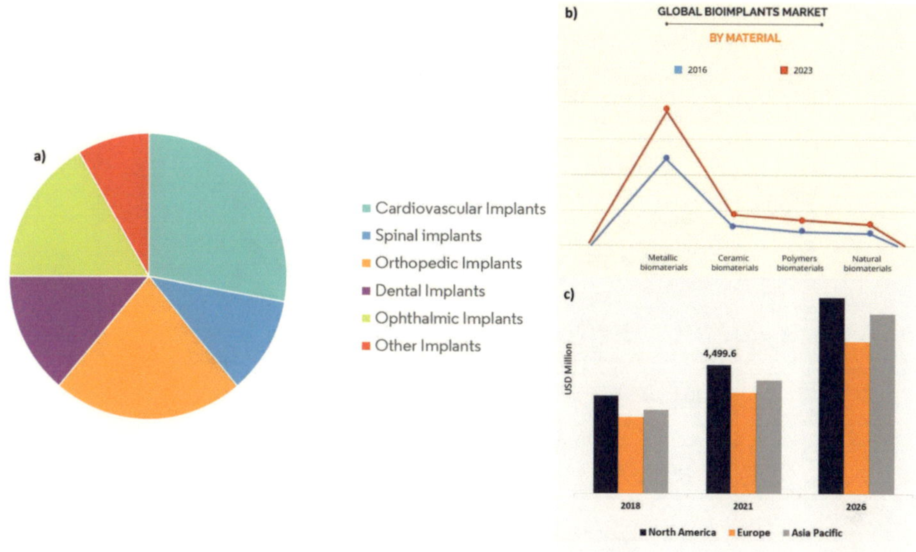

Figure 1.
Bioimplants market share by (a) type of implant, (b) implant material, and (c) region [13–15].

The metallic and medical alloy industry is mostly dominated by permanent implants such as titanium, cobalt chromium, and stainless steel. However, emerging biodegradable materials like Mg-based alloys compete with orthopedic implants and cardiovascular stents. They serve as improved substitutes for previously used biodegradable polymeric devices due to their load-bearing capacity [16]. Other biodegradable metallic materials such as Zn- and Fe-based alloys have not been as successful as their Mg counterpart in application. Mg alloys are currently being developed for various biomedical applications and degrade at different rates to match specific needs.

2. Microstructural and mechanical properties

Magnesium has a hexagonal closed pack (hcp) crystal structure, which is beneficial for strength but detrimental to ductility. This is because an hcp crystal structure does not possess enough independent slip systems required for dislocation movement and uniform deformation. Introducing other alloying elements into magnesium can alter its texture and improve mechanical behavior. Several magnesium-based alloys with biodegradable and biocompatible alloying elements have been investigated for biomedical applications. Most of the studies are focused on improving mechanical performance and combating high initial degradation rates, localized degradation, and hydrogen evolution. For instance, addition of rare earth (RE) metals or manganese (Mn) improves strength, zirconia (Zr) provides grain refinement and increases corrosion resistance, zinc (Zn) also increases corrosion resistance and strength, whereas calcium (Ca) reduces oxidation and allow for easy rollability. Lithium (Li) is one element that stands out because it transforms the hcp crystal structure of magnesium to a body-centered cubic (bcc), thereby increasing the ductility of the alloy and, in some cases, making it superplastic. In addition, Li also provides very good corrosion resistance by developing a uniform oxide surface coating. **Figure 2** shows a plot of the ultimate tensile strength and elongation of some researched Mg-Li-based

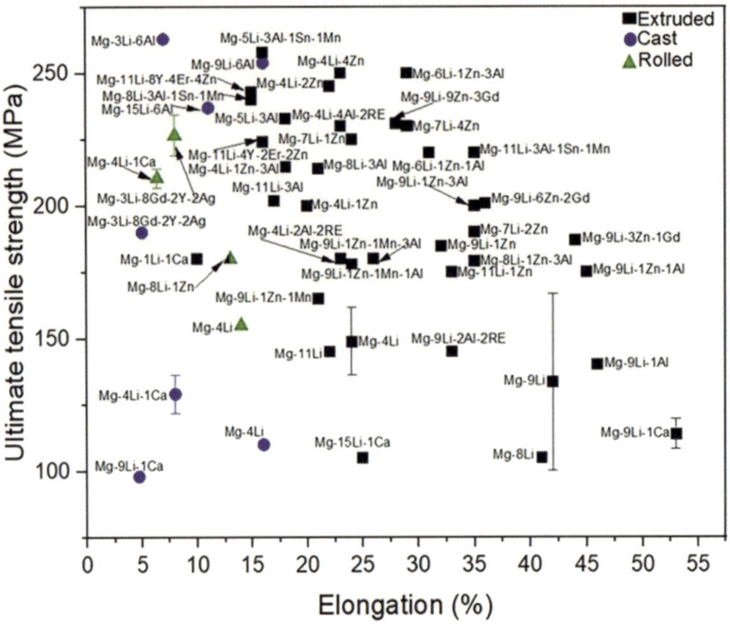

Figure 2.
Ultimate tensile strength vs. elongation for select Mg-Li-based alloys.

alloys. Careful introduction of metallic elements, both the choice of elements and the alloying percentages, in a fashion that will enhance both mechanical and degradation performance is of optimum importance.

When lithium is added to magnesium, it forms a solid solution of α-Mg up to ~5.3 wt.% Li, after which dual phase α-Mg and β-Li coexist in equilibrium up to 10.7 wt.% Li. Further increase in Li content results in phase transformation into a single β-Li phase, as shown in the Mg-Li binary phase diagram of **Figure 3**. These changes in crystal structure yield corresponding improvements in room temperature ductility but can negatively impact mechanical strength.

2.1 Crystalline phases and phase transformations

The crystalline phases present in an alloy makeup its microstructure; they determine crystal structures, textures, and deformation behavior. In addition, phase transformations such as those induced by the addition of Li to Mg also impact the mechanical and corrosion properties of the alloy. In a study of Mg-xLi-1Zn-0.5Ca (x = 0, 4, 8, 11) cast alloys [18], x-ray diffractograms shown in **Figure 4** revealed that the predominant peaks for alloys with 0 and 4 wt.% Li (L0 and L4) were those of magnesium. Minor diffraction peaks of Mg_2Ca and $Ca_2Mg_6Zn_3$ phases were also detected. For the alloy with 8 wt.% Li (L8), peaks of both magnesium and lithium phases, as well as the secondary Mg_2Ca phase, were detected, whereas the alloy with 11 wt.% Li (L11) displayed a predominant lithium phase with a secondary Mg_2Ca phase. The primary crystalline phase of both alloys L0 and L4 had the hcp structure; that of L8 had a combination of hcp and bcc while L11 had only bcc. The primary crystalline phases of these alloys agree with those of the Mg-Li binary phase diagram.

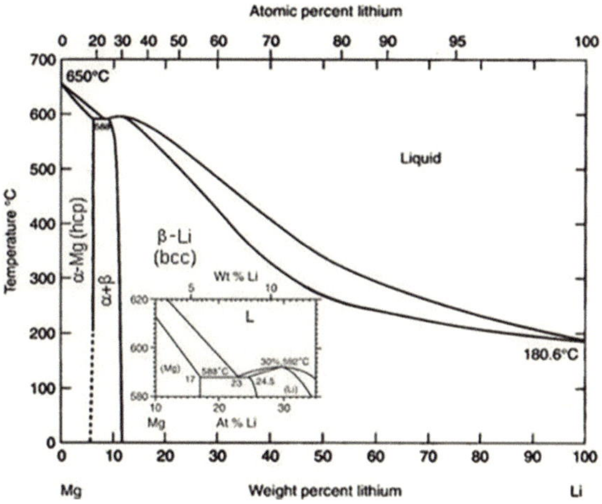

Figure 3.
Equilibrium binary phase diagram of magnesium and lithium [17].

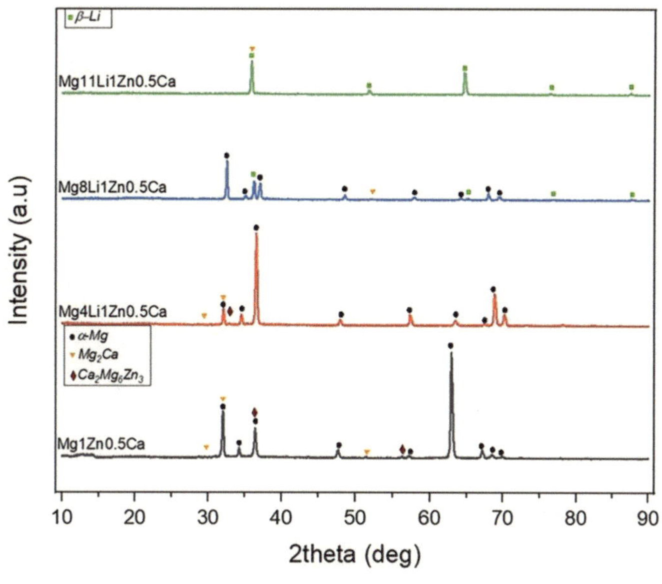

Figure 4.
X-ray diffractograms of Mg-xLi-1Zn-0.5Ca alloys.

2.2 Strength and ductility

Strength and ductility are two fundamental properties that are assessed for biomedical alloys. A tensile or compressive test can be used to determine the yield and ultimate strengths, and elongation of alloys. Mechanical property requirements may vary for specific implant applications, but alloys are usually expected to have a minimum strength and ductility to enable easy processing and fabrication of devices. Other mechanical tests that could be assessed include hardness, strain hardening, fatigue strength, and wear resistance.

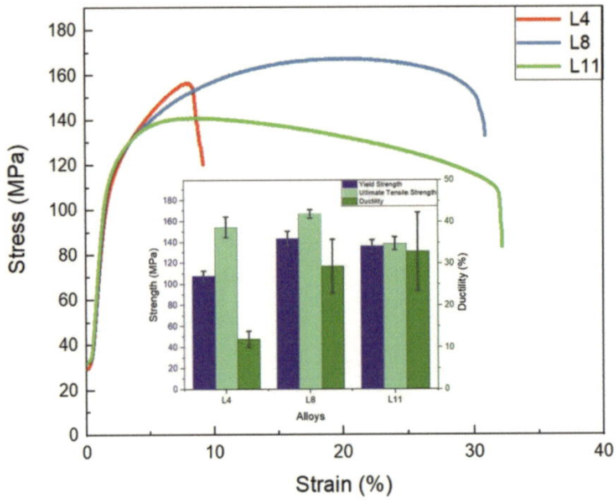

Figure 5.
Stress–strain curves and tensile parameters of Mg-xLi-1Zn-0.5Ca alloys.

Tensile test data shown in **Figure 5** shows how Li content affects the strength and ductility of alloys, as reported in Section 2.1. Increasing the Li content progressively increases the ductility of the alloy across the three phases, but the strength is maximum in the dual phases. Although strength can be attributed to several factors such as grain size, presence, and distribution of secondary phases, here, the alloying content and proportion of both the α-Mg and β-Li phases also play a role. Several thermomechanical techniques such as extrusion, equal channel angular pressing (ECAP), and friction stir process (FSP) improve the strength and ductility of Mg alloys, but Mg-Li alloys tend to possess very good elastic and superplasticity, especially in the duplex phase [19].

The mechanical properties of biodegradable implants can be tuned by alloying, thermomechanical processing, surface modification, polymer coating, and other such treatments. The initial mechanical properties should account for the effect of biodegradation, such that the implant devices are able to provide the required mechanical support throughout the healing time.

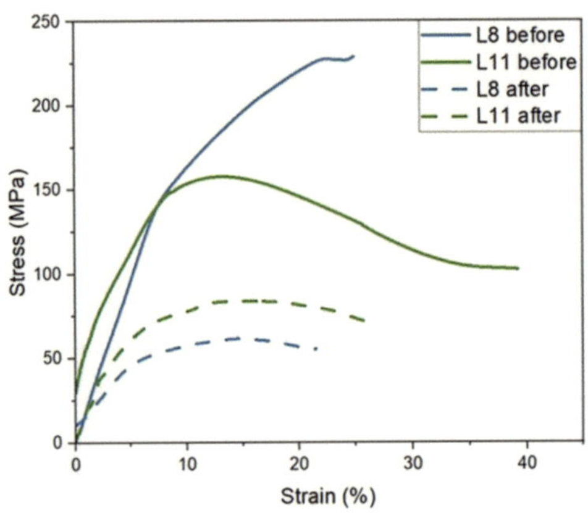

Figure 6.
Stress–strain curve of Mg-8Li-1Zn-0.5Ca (L8) and Mg-11Li-1Zn-0.5Ca (L11) before and after accelerated durability tests.

Figure 6 demonstrates the changes in mechanical strength with degradation time for the L8 and L11 alloys. Specimens of these alloys were subject to accelerated durability tests in saline solution via pulsatile loading with the average regular human heart rate of 72 beats per minute (bpm) for a specified time. The average stress-strain plots after compression tests revealed a higher maximum stress of ~228 MPa for the L8 alloy compared to the L11 alloy (~158 MPa) before durability testing. In contrast, the L11 possessed a higher maximum strength of ~79 MPa compared to L8 (57 MPa) after pulsatile loading. This represents about 50% and 75% loss in strength for alloys of L8 and L11, respectively, after about 3 months implantation period.

3. Electrochemical behavior

Generally, corrosion is unwanted in engineering and science applications. However, in the case of biodegradable implants, controlled degradation can revolutionize biomedical implantation. The biodegradation of materials refers to the gradual removal and atomic disintegration of materials in a biological environment. This process is characterized by electrochemical reactions and can be studied by the corrosion processes of metals. Corrosion normally occurs at a rate determined by equilibrium between opposing electrochemical reactions. An anodic reaction occurs when the metal is oxidized, releasing electrons into the metal. A cathodic reaction is in which a solution species (often O_2 or H^+) consumes the electrons released from the metal. When these two reactions are in equilibrium, the flow of electrons from each reaction is balanced, and no net electron flow (electrical current) occurs. The two reactions can take place on one metal or on two dissimilar metals (or metal sites) that are electrically connected.

The composition and strength of the electrolyte or environment in which the material is housed plays an important role in its degradation behavior. Degradation behavior can be assessed *in vivo*, where the material under test is implanted within a living organism, or *in vitro*, where the materials are tested in simulated biological conditions. *In vivo* testing provides more accurate conditions for assessing implant materials but does not allow the variation of single parameters within the study.

Mg alloys degrade in aqueous environment to produce Mg hydroxide ($Mg(OH)_2$) and hydrogen gas (H_2) with an overall electrochemical reaction shown in Eq. (1). When chloride concentration rises above 30 mmol/l, Mg hydroxide starts to convert into highly soluble Mg chloride [20]. Low hydrogen over potential enables hydrogen evolution and galvanic corrosion, especially when secondary phases are present. It is important to note that although precipitation strengthening and grain refinement improve strength and ductility, care should be taken to prevent localized degradation resulting from galvanic pairs:

$$Mg + 2H_2O \rightarrow Mg(OH)_2 + H_2 \tag{1}$$

Implant degradation is dependent on several factors such as material composition, device geometry, and environment. The rate of electrochemical reaction and formation and stability of oxide films also depend on reduction and oxidation reactions, time of exposure, and temperature. The corrosive environment of the human body is dependent on the composition of blood and other body fluids, as well as the body temperature. Furthermore, the effect of protein adsorption depends on metal/biomolecule combinations and can promote or reduce degradation rates for different cases [21].

3.1 Factors affecting corrosion behavior

The most important requirement of a biodegradable implant is – its degradation properties in a specific biological environment, which are influenced by various intrinsic and extrinsic factors. Intrinsic factors include chemical composition, microstructure, surface energy, wettability, thickness, and stability of the passivating oxide film. Extrinsic factors include temperature, pH, dissolved oxygen content, amino acids, biomolecules, and chloride ions in the surrounding environment [22]. Tissue fluids within the human body present a very corrosive environment for implant devices. In addition to inorganic species in body fluid, different types of biomolecules and cells may attach to the implant surface and affect its surface chemistry. The regeneration of a passivating oxide film is delayed since the concentration of dissolved oxygen in body fluids is approximately one-fourth of that in air. Additionally, the concentration of Cl^- ions in serum and interstitial fluid is 113 and 117 mEq/L, respectively [22]. Cl^- ions induce pitting corrosion at sites where the passive film is broken. This is followed by the propagation of the pit, at a rate that occasionally increases with time, because of the increasing acidity inside the pit.

3.1.1 Corrosion kinetics

Electrochemical reactions have been identified to proceed in a linear, parabolic, or logarithmic fashion [2]. The parabolic rate law is attributed to the diffusion of solvent ions through a porous film produced during the corrosion reaction, thus retarding its rate. The rate-determining step is diffusion through a passivating film; thickness of film increases in proportion to the extent of corrosion. For linear oxidation, the rate of oxidation or corrosion generally depends on the pore volume and the "tortuosity" of the pores as well as the film thickness. This is because highly porous, poorly adherent, and fractured non-protective oxide layers do not retard ionic diffusion and the rate of corrosion.

3.1.2 Oxide formation and pilling-Bedworth ratio

Electrochemical redox reactions involve the transfer of electrons and change in oxidation states of elements present within the alloy. Oxide formation is constrained by reaction thermodynamics with a driving force given by the potential difference of redox half-reactions. Oxides with minimum energy of formation are preferentially formed, and a lower enthalpy of formation is indicative of greater chemical stability [23]. However, the effective driving force of metal oxidation reduces as the oxide grows because of potential distribution [24]. The Pilling–Bedworth ratio (PBR) is used to describe the volume ratio and stress states of metals and their oxide films. Generally, a ratio less than 1 is indicative of a thin oxide coating with tensile stresses, which offers poor protection, and a ratio greater than 1 indicates the oxides are denser with compressive stresses and offer more protection. Higher ratios indicate growth in stress, and beyond 2, large compressive stresses result in cracking and spallation of the oxide film. The PBR of compounds can be calculated using Eq. (2):

$$PBR = \frac{M_{oxide} \times \rho_{metal}}{n \times M_{metal} \times \rho_{oxide}} \tag{2}$$

Compound	MgO	CaO	ZnO	Li_2O	LiOH	$Mg(OH)_2$	$MgCO_3$	$CaCO_3$	Li_2CO_3
PBR	0.80	0.64	1.59	0.57	1.26	1.80	2.04	1.43	1.35

Table 2.
Pilling–Bedworth ratios of select compounds.

where M and ρ are the respective molecular weights and densities, and n is the number of metal atoms in the oxide molecule (**Table 2**).

3.2 Electrochemical methods for accessing corrosion behavior

Electrochemical techniques are ideal for the study of corrosion processes because they provide accelerated corrosion rates as opposed to the conventional weight loss/gain method that requires an extended period for measurements. In electrochemical studies, a metal sample of a known surface area is used to model a redox reaction occurring on the surface of a metal immersed in an electrolyte. The potential between the metal and a reference electrode is varied using a potentiostat, and the current flowing through a counter electrode is measured as a function of potential. The corrosion rate is governed by Faraday's law given in Eq. (3):

$$Q = \frac{nFW}{M} \tag{3}$$

where Q is the total current (coulombs), n is the number of electrons involved in the electrochemical reaction, W is the weight of the metal (grams), M is the molecular weight (grams), and F is the Faraday's constant (96,485 coulombs/mole).

Accelerated corrosion tests can be used to assess the bio-electrochemical, electro-physicochemical, and electrochemical degradation of Mg alloys within a specific environment. Usually, a potentiostat connected to a three-electrode setup with a standard, counter, and working electrode (the alloy under test) is used to measure the corrosion rate. Different types of accelerated corrosion tests are available to study the degradation behavior of bioresorbable alloys such as potentiodynamic polarization, linear polarization, cyclic voltammetry, and electrochemical impedance spectroscopy.

3.2.1 Potentiodynamic polarization

Potentiodynamic polarization (PP) uses a wide range DC potential to scan the alloy, causing redox reactions and generating corrosion current. The polarization curve can be used to determine the corrosion rate of the alloys from the Tafel slope and according to Faraday's law in Eq. (4). This technique requires the corrosion potential to remain the same during the measurement to ensure that the applied overvoltage is known. When using the open circuit voltage (Eoc) for polarization, it is imperative to allow sufficient time for the electrochemical double layer to achieve a steady state so that Eoc is stabilized:

$$C.R. = \frac{I_{corr} \times K \times E.W}{A \times \rho} \tag{4}$$

where K is a constant, Icorr is the corrosion current, E.W is the equivalent weight, A is the exposed area, and r is the density of the alloy.

3.2.2 Electrochemical impedance spectroscopy

Electrochemical impedance spectroscopy (EIS) measures the response of the alloy under test to AC perturbation. In this technique, it is assumed that the following conditions are met.

1. The response of the system to external excitation can be described by linear differential equations.

2. The system is stable and returns to its previous state after the removal of the external excitation.

3. There is no response before the excitation.

4. The response to excitation has a relationship that is finite.

For an applied signal, Et, which depends on time and frequency, there is a response signal. According to Ohm's law, an impedance, Z, can be calculated and represented in terms of magnitude and phase shift angle. The measured data resulting from the development of a potential difference between the electric double layer is modeled to an equivalent electrical circuit.

In EIS, the impedance of the corroding metal (working electrode) due to an applied sinusoidal potential change (AC voltage) is analyzed as a function of frequency ω. At each frequency, the resulting sinusoidal current waveform and the applied potential are out-of-phase by phase angle (θ), whereas the current amplitude is inversely proportional to the impedance of the interface. The electrochemical impedance, Z (ω), is the frequency-dependent proportionality factor in the relationship between the voltage signal and the current response, as given in Eq. (5)

$$Z(\omega) = E(\omega) / i(\omega). \tag{5}$$

where E is the voltage signal, E = E0 sin (ω t); i is the current density, i = i0 sin (ω t + θ); Z is the impedance (ohm/cm^2); and t is the time (seconds).

The impedance is a complex number described by the frequency-dependent modulus, |Z|, and the phase angle, θ, or, otherwise, by the real and imaginary components, Z′, and Z″ [25]. In electrochemical impedance analysis, three different types of plots are commonly used, including two bode plots, which show impedance and phase angle against frequency. The third is a Nyquist plot, which shows complex plane Z″ vs. Z′, and the capacitive arc provides an estimate of the corrosion resistance of the material. The relative diameter of the arc is directly proportional to the charge transfer resistance or polarization resistance (Rp). Thus, an increase in semicircular diameter corresponds to an increase in corrosion resistance.

It should be noted that since real electrochemical processes hardly show pure capacitance, during EIS analysis, the non-ideal response of the corrosion system is represented by a constant phase element to obtain accurate impedance values. These are due to geometric distributions, such as surface inhomogeneities and porosity of the electrode.

Figure 7 shows plots from electrochemical impedance spectroscopy of Mg-*x*Li-1Zn-0.5Ca. The Nyquist plot exhibits different capacitive arcs for the different alloys with relative diameters indicative of their corrosion resistance. The polarization resistance which is clearly seen in the lower frequency region of the impedance bode plot, demonstrates whether an electrode/alloy is reactive or blocking. Furthermore, changes observed in the phase angles illustrate the distinct dielectric behavior of each alloy. In addition to alloy composition, thermomechanical processing plays a major role in degradation kinetics. For example, FSP of dual-phase Mg-Li-Al-Zn alloys resulted in a synergetic strength ductility corrosion optimization by a combinatory contribution of fine grains and nanosized precipitated which inhibited microgalvanic

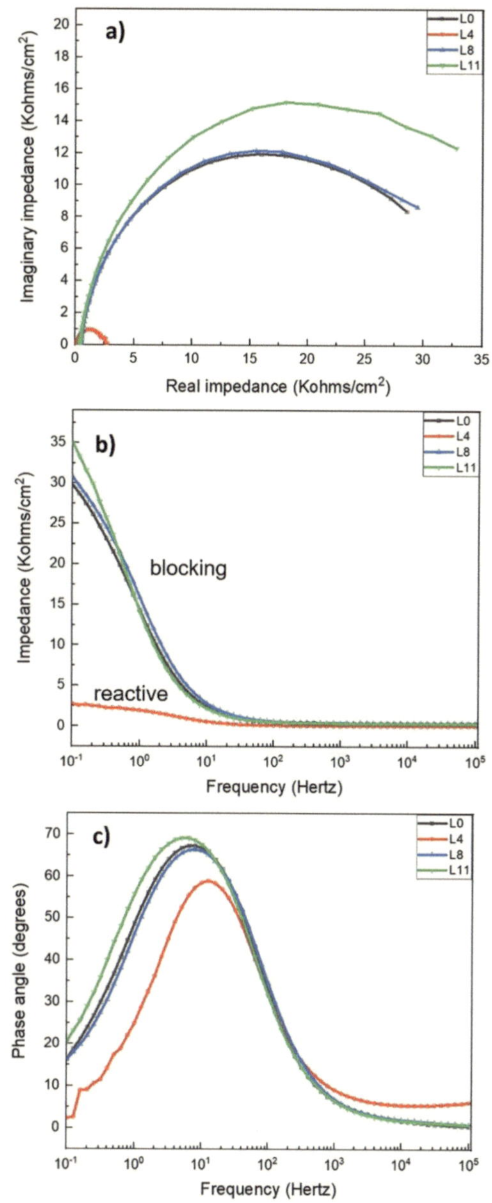

Figure 7.
Electrochemical impedance plots (a) Nyquist plot, (b) impedance bode plot, and (c) phase angle bode plot of Mg-xLi-1Zn-0.5Ca alloys.

corrosion [26]. A study on optimized Mg-Li-Al-Zr-Y extruded alloys [27] showed decreasing dissolution kinetics as we move from water quenched (WQ) to artificially aged WQ (WQA) to cold rolled WQA (WQAR), as such optimization is required to achieve the best candidate alloys decreasing anodic kinetics compared to pure Mg. The difference in electrochemical response is dependent on the microstructure of the alloy. As the alloy moves from hcp to hcp + bcc to fully bcc, oxide formation, and surface film coverage varies. In the single hcp phase, the surface protection is made up of Mg oxides and hydroxides, which offer poor coverage. However, in the dual phase, there is a development of more stable Li oxide and carbonate, but in the fully bcc phase, complete coverage is achieved with a uniform thick Li carbonate outer layer.

3.3 Immersion tests for accessing corrosion behavior

Immersion tests require immersing the alloy in physiological medium for a specific amount of time. This is important because it provides the opportunity to monitor the degradation process and provide direct observation of the alloy at specific times. The hydrodynamic condition of the test setup, among other things, influences the degradation behavior of the alloys. Immersion tests can thus be classified as static, semi-static, or dynamic. For static immersion, degradation occurs in the same media for the specified test duration. On the other hand, dynamic immersion involves the constant flow of the immersion media. Finally, semi-static immersion allows for periodic changes in immersion media.

Semi-static immersion provides a good balance between the static and dynamic test setups, good volume-to-area ratios, and immersion time to avoid distortion of test

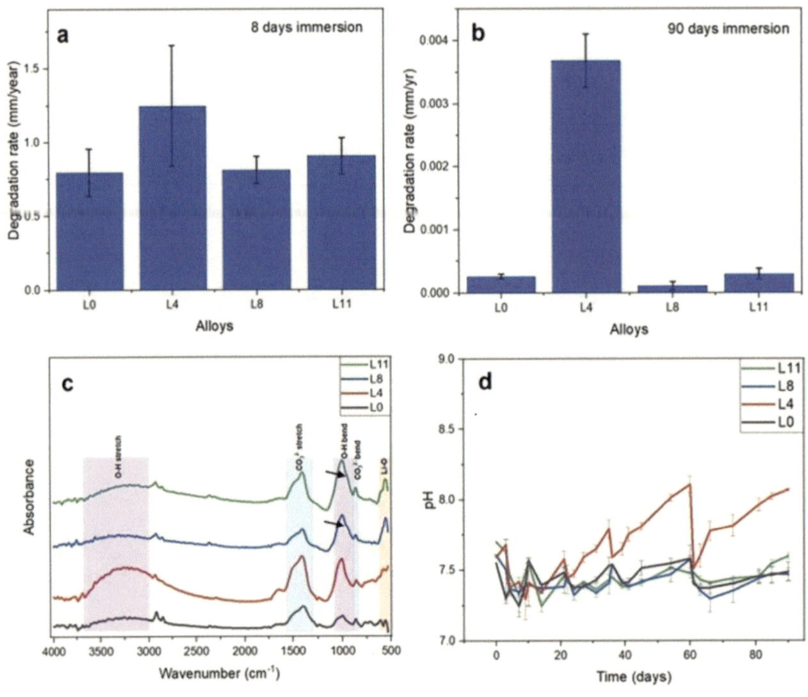

Figure 8.
Degradation rates of Mg-xLi-1Zn-0.5Ca alloys after immersion for (a) 8 days, (b) 90 days, (c) FTIR spectra of degraded alloys, and (d) pH measurements after 90 days.

conditions. In addition, the periodic media changes mimic fluid changes at implantation sites and prevent passivation of Mg alloys at elevated pH values. For semi-static immersion, mass transfer is controlled by migration, diffusion, and a certain degree of convection generated by hydrogen evolution [28].

The determination of corrosion rate can be achieved by volume loss, mass loss, and hydrogen evolution. These methods can generate different results due to testing and measurement limitations such as incomplete removal of corrosion materials during mass loss calculation. The volume loss method can be used both in vivo and in vitro while the hydrogen evolution method can be carried out using a eudiometer system which has to be properly calibrated and well-sealed to avoid the escape of hydrogen atoms. However, mass and volume loss methods have provided consistent results [29]. Chemical cleaning using reagents such as chromic acid is recommended for corrosion product removal to attain uniform weight measurement.

Semi-static immersion on Mg-Li-based alloys reported in Section 2.1 for mass loss after 8 and 90 days is shown in **Figure 8**. A reduction in degradation rate for L8 and L11 is recorded with increased immersion time, with L8 and L4 having the lowest and highest degradation rates, respectively. Scanning electron microscopy micrographs show the post-immersion morphology of the alloys after 8 days in **Figure 9**. There is the presence of flakes and multidimensional cracks, and L0 exhibited some islands ($Ca_2Mg_6Zn_3$ rich region) surrounded by Mg-rich zones. Furthermore, Mg-rich pits demarcated by the Mg_2Ca region were observed. Alloy L4 also displayed pits with high oxide content on the periphery and showed increased pH indicative of an accelerated electrochemical reaction (see **Figure 8d**). The formation of oxides of

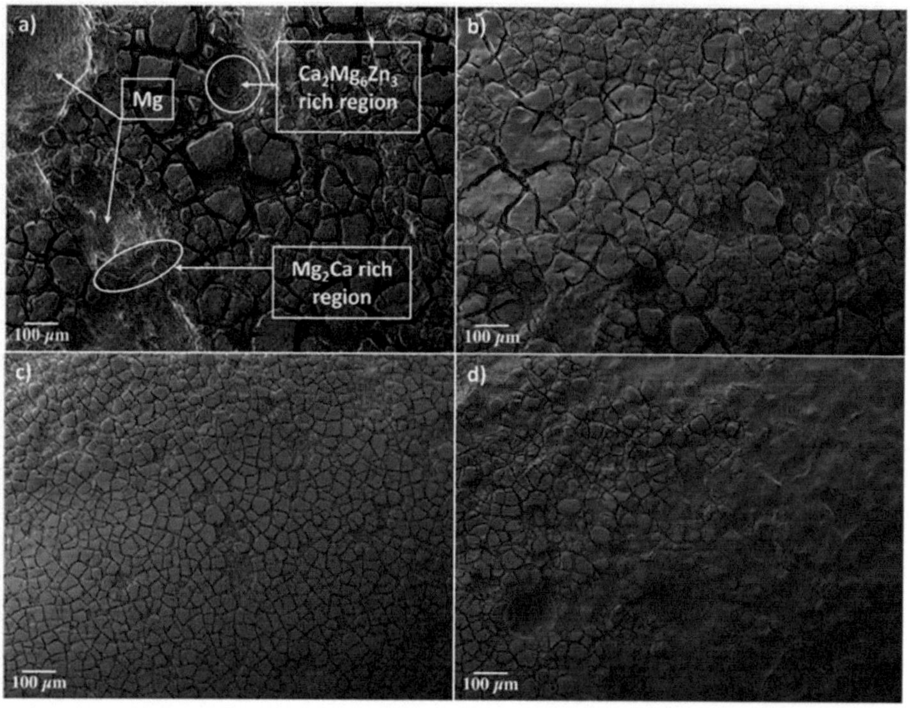

Figure 9.
Post-immersion morphology of (a) Mg-1Zn-0.5Ca, (b) Mg-4Li-1Zn-0.5Ca, (c) Mg-8Li-1Zn-0.5Ca, and (d) Mg-11Li-1Zn-0.5Ca alloys after 8 days.

MgO, Li_2O, and CaO with PBR <1 is responsible for surface cracking resulting from tensile stresses in the oxide films. This allows the penetration of H_2O and CO_2, leading to the formation of more stable hydroxide and carbonate films. Oxides formed on alloy surfaces can be assessed with tools such as Fourier transform infrared spectroscopy (FTIR), as shown in **Figure 8c**. The formation of more stable oxides reduced degradation kinetics for Mg-Li alloys in the dual and β-Li phases due to the formation of a passive Li_2CO_3 film.

A proper electrochemical assessment of biodegradable implant materials cannot be overemphasized. This is because uncontrolled degradation can lead to pitting, which alters the microstructural composition and mechanical properties of the alloy. Furthermore, when electrochemical redox reaction occurs at an accelerated rate, as is the case with localized degradation, there is a larger amount of ionic dissolution. Such uncontrolled release may result in tissue overload and cytotoxicity.

4. Biocompatibility

Biocompatibility is fundamental for any type of materials intended for use within the human body. When devices are implanted either for diagnosis or therapeutic cases, certain reactions can be generated because of the interaction between the body and the foreign material. These reactions are dependent on the physiochemical properties of the implanted device as well as the implantation site. Generally, the biocompatibility of implant materials is influenced by their surface properties such as surface morphology, chemical composition, surface charge, corrosion rate, thickness, and the nature of the passivation layers.

It is important that metallic implants are biocompatible and non-toxic. In addition, bioresorbable implants also need to degrade in a fashion that does not cause tissue overload arising from very fast degradation. Biocompatibility analysis can be conducted *in vivo* (as in the case of animal studies) or in vitro using cell lines. It is essential that the implant materials are assessed with cell lines that are related to their intended implantation sites. Materials developed for applications such as cardiovascular use can be assessed with endothelial cell lines, whereas those for orthopedic use can be assessed with osteoblast cell lines.

Different types of assessments can be employed for biocompatibility studies. Commonly used tests include wettability, cytotoxicity, hemocompatibility, and antibacterial responses.

4.1 Wettability

Wettability is a property which influences material-cellular interaction and can be determined by contact angle measurements. It involves measuring the angle a drop of solvent makes with the solid material substrate. Contact angle measurements can be used to determine hydrophilic or hydrophobic properties, surface adhesion, energy, and adsorption via several methods such as sessile or pendant drop. The contact angle differs for various solvents such as water, ethylene glycol, etc., and is dependent on the surface finish and characteristics of the substrate material. Equilibrium contact angle, θ, can be determined from Young's equation:

$$\gamma_{lv} cos\theta = \gamma_{sv} - \gamma_{sl} \tag{6}$$

where γ_{sv} and γ_{lv} are the surface energy of the solid and liquid, respectively, and γ_{sl} is solid–liquid interfacial energy.

4.2 Cytotoxicity

A cytotoxicity assessment makes it possible to investigate to what extent a foreign material can coexist with living tissues without causing any toxic effect. Even when bioresorbable implant materials are designed from non-toxic elements, their biocompatibility responses should be assessed as degradation and wear rate can also result in toxicity [30]. A cytotoxicity analysis involves exposing human cells to a test material either directly or indirectly to its dissolved constituent ions to ensure that the implant will not generate high concentrations of ions that can harm surrounding tissues when implanted.

Figure 10 shows cytotoxicity analysis of Mg-xLi-1Zn-0.5Ca alloys on human umbilical vein endothelial cells (HUVEC) with different incubation times. There is increased metabolic activity and cell proliferation with increased incubation time. Other studies on cytotoxicity analysis for Mg-(3.5, 6.5) Li-(0.5, 2, 4) Zn alloys

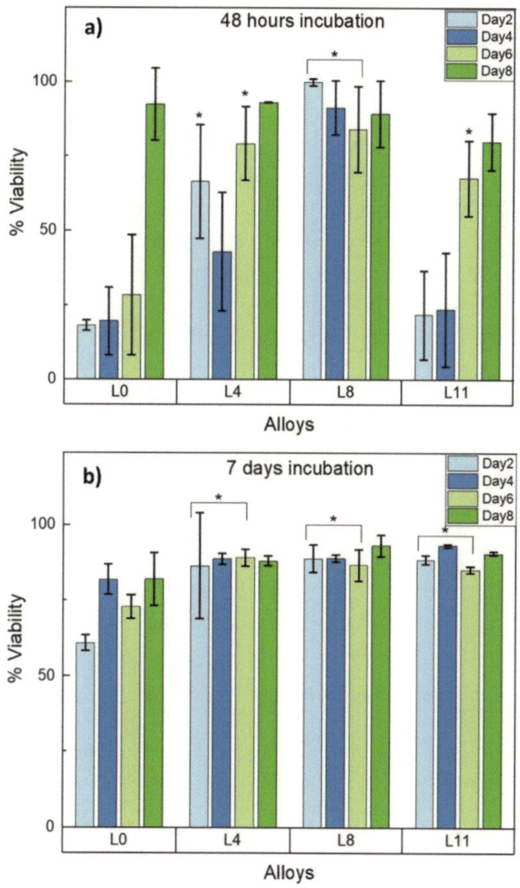

Figure 10.
Cell viability responses of Mg-xLi-1Zn-0.5Ca alloys on HUVEC after (a) 48 hours and (b) 7 days incubation period.

conducted on vascular smooth muscle cells (VSMC) and HUVEC [31] showed that apoptosis was more prevalent in VSMC given the pH and ion concentration of extracts used for the culture. This shows that significant changes in responses can be achieved with different cell lines.

4.3 Hemocompatibility

Hemocompatibility can provide insight into interactions that might trigger activation, secretion, adherence and aggregation of platelets, coagulation, and immunological responses when an implant material encounters blood [32, 33]. It plays a major role in thrombogenicity and is dependent on material's surface properties. Understanding blood interactions is important because they eventually lead to the formation of a thrombus. Thrombosis can be dangerous when a clot forms within a vessel and cuts off supply, which is a leading clinical complication for stent failure. A hemocompatibility assessment investigates the affinity of blood and its constituents to an implant material, which can be measured using platelet adhesion analysis.

5. Conclusion

The development of functional and safe bioresorbable Mg alloys will be useful in the fabrication of temporary implant devices for both orthopedic and cardiovascular applications.

1. Mg-Li-Zn-Ca alloys, as an example of Mg-Li-based implant material, exhibited enhanced ductility and strength, which are important mechanical properties required not only for a medical device's in-service application but also good formability that favors ease in manufacturing.

2. The alloys exhibited uniform degradation behavior, which is a very important property for temporary metallic implants such as cardiovascular stents, plates, and screws because it mitigates against early loss of mechanical integrity associated with localized or pitting degradation.

3. Increased cell viability and metabolic activity imply their biocompatibility and nontoxicity, which will mitigate clinical complications and instill confidence in the deployment of magnesium-based prostheses.

Author details

Chiamaka Okafor and Norman Munroe*
Florida International University, Miami, USA

*Address all correspondence to: munroen@fiu.edu

References

[1] Agrawal CM. Reconstructing the human body using biomaterials. JOM [Internet]. 1998;**50**(1):31-35. Available from: https://link.springer.com/article/10.1007/s11837-998-0064-5. [Accessed: July 18, 2023]

[2] Gill PKS. Assessment of Biodegradable Magnesium Alloys for Enhanced Mechanical and Biocompatible Properties. USA: Florida International University; 2012

[3] Yunchang X. Deformation Mechanism and Surface Modification of Biomedical Magnesium Alloy. Hong Kong: City University of Hong Kong; 2009

[4] Aljihmani L, Alic L, Boudjemline Y, Hijazi ZM, Mansoor B, Serpedin E, et al. Magnesium-based Bioresorbable stent materials: Review of reviews. Journal of Bio- and Tribo-Corrosion. 2019;**5**:26

[5] Werkhoven RJ, Sillekens WH, Van Lieshout JBJM. Processing aspects of magnesium alloy stent tube. In: Magnesium Technology. Cham: Springer; 2011. pp. 419-424

[6] Peuster M, Beerbaum P, Bach FW, Hauser H. Are resorbable implants about to become a reality? Cardiology in the Young. 2006;**16**:107-116

[7] Poncin P, Millet C, Chevy J, Proft J. Comparing and optimizing Co-Cr tubing for stent applications. In: Medical Device Materials II - Proceedings of the Materials and Processes for Medical Devices Conference, USA. Vol. 2005. 2004. pp. 279-283

[8] AMP R. Magnesium in health and disease. In: Astrid S, Sigel H, Sigel RKO, editors. Interrelations between Essential Metal Ions and Human Diseases. Dordrecht: Springer Netherlands; 2013. pp. 49-79

[9] National Academy Press, Disaster Prevention and Management. Vol. 23. No. 8(4). United Kingdom: Emerald Group Publishing; 1999. p. 23

[10] Institute of Medicine. Dietary Reference Intakes for Vitamin a, Vitamin K, Arsenic, Boron, Chromium, Copper, Iodine, Iron, Manganese, Molybdenum, Nickel, Silicon, Vanadium, and Zinc. Institute of Medicine. USA: The National Academy Press; 2001

[11] Gill P, Munroe N, Datye A. Synthesis, characterization and mechanical properties of biodegradable magnesium alloys. Emerging. Materials Research. 2013;**2**(EMR 1):45-52

[12] Dey K. Bioimplants Market Trends, Growth and Size Analysis. USA: Market Research Future; 2023

[13] Prateeksha K. Bioimplants Market. USA: Allied Market Research; 2018

[14] Reports and Data. Metal Implant and Medical Alloys Market. USA: Reports and Data; 2020 (RND_002472)

[15] Mordor intelligence [Internet]. Bio-Implants Market. Growth, Trends and Forecast. India: Mordor intelligence; 2017

[16] Lyon P. The Benefits of Magnesium Alloys for Medical Implants. United Kingdom: Medical Design Briefs; 2017

[17] Pezda J, Białobrzeski A. Registration of melting and crystallization process of ultra-light weight MgLi12,5 alloy with use of ATND method. Archives of Foundry Engineering. 2012;**12**(2):143-146

[18] Okafor C, Datye A, Zhang S, Schwarz UD, Cai Y, Munroe N. Development and biomaterial characterization of Mg-Li-Zn-Ca alloys. Materials Today Communications. 2022;**33**(1-13):104999

[19] Savaedi Z, Motallebi R, Mirzadeh H, Mehdinavaz Aghdam R, Mahmudi R. Superplasticity of Fine-Grained Magnesium Alloys for Biomedical Applications: A Comprehensive Review. Vol. 27. Elsevier Ltd: Current Opinion in Solid State and Materials Science; 2023

[20] Witte F, Hort N, Vogt C, Cohen S, Kainer KU, Willumeit R, et al. Degradable biomaterials based on magnesium corrosion. Current Opinion in Solid State & Materials Science [Internet]. 2008;**12**(5):63-72. Available from: https://www.sciencedirect.com/science/article/pii/S1359028609000357

[21] Virtanen S, Milošev I, Gomez-Barrena E, Trebše R, Salo J, Konttinen YT. Special modes of corrosion under physiological and simulated physiological conditions. Acta Biomaterialia. 2008;**4**(3):468-476

[22] Haider W. Enhanced Biocompatibility of NiTi (Nitinol) Via Surface Treatment and Alloying. USA: Florida International University; 2010

[23] Zeng RC, Sun L, Zheng YF, Cui HZ, Han EH. Corrosion and characterisation of dual phase Mg-Li-Ca alloy in Hank's solution: The influence of microstructural features. Corrosion Science [Internet]. 2014;**79**:69-82. DOI: 10.1016/j.corsci.2013.10.028

[24] Momeni M, Wren JC. A mechanistic model for oxide growth and dissolution during corrosion of Cr-containing alloys. Faraday Discussions. 2015;**180**:113-135

[25] Silman H. Corrosion and corrosion control: An introduction to corrosion science and engineering. British Corrosion Journal [Internet]. 1972;**7**:98. Available from: https://api.semanticscholar.org/CorpusID:135548984

[26] Zhu Y, Chen G, Zhou Y, Shi Q, Zhou M. Achieving synergistic strength-ductility-corrosion optimization in Mg-Li-Al-Zn alloy via cross-pass friction stir processing. Journal of Alloys and Compounds. 2023;**959**:170581

[27] Xu W, Birbilis N, Sha G, Wang Y, Daniels JE, Xiao Y, et al. A high-specific-strength and corrosion-resistant magnesium alloy. Nature Materials [Internet]. 2015;**14**(12):1229-1235. Available from: https://www.nature.com/articles/nmat4435

[28] Gonzalez J, Hou RQ, Nidadavolu EPS, Willumeit-Römer R, Feyerabend F. Magnesium degradation under physiological conditions – Best practice. Bioactive Materials. 2018;**3**(2):174-185

[29] Liu L, Gebresellasie K, Collins B, Zhang H, Xu Z, Sankar J, et al. Degradation rates of pure zinc, magnesium, and magnesium alloys measured by volume loss, mass loss, and hydrogen evolution. Applied Sciences [Internet]. 2018;**8**:1459. DOI: 10.3390/app8091459

[30] Hanawa T. Evaluation techniques of metallic biomaterials in vitro. Science and Technology of Advanced Materials. 2002;**3**(4):289-295

[31] Liu Y, Wu Y, Bian D, Gao S, Leeflang S, Guo H, et al. Study on the Mg-Li-Zn ternary alloy system with improved mechanical properties, good degradation performance and different responses to cells. Acta Biomaterialia

[Internet]. 2017;**62**:418-433. DOI: 10.1016/j.actbio.2017.08.021

[32] Peek GJ, Firmin RK. The inflammatory and coagulative response to prolonged extracorporeal membrane oxygenation. ASAIO Journal [Internet]. 1999;**45**(4):250-263. Available from: https://api.semanticscholar.org/CorpusID:41675889

[33] Amruthaluri S. An Investigation on Biocompatibility of Bio-Absorbable Polymer Coated Magnesium Alloys [Internet]. USA: Florida International University; 2014. Available from: http://digitalcommons.fiu.edu/etd/1283

Chapter 3

Hydroxyapatite Composites in Tissue Engineering

Senny Thomas Parackal, Jose Paul, Johnson Dlima, Puthiya Veettil Darshana, Alenya Mary Pyas, Chamalayil AbdulRahman Syed Mohammed Jiffry and Sruthi K. Nair

Abstract

In the last few decades, material sciences, particularly tissue engineering, have advanced significantly. Biomaterials, including bioceramics, such as hydroxyapatite and bioglass, have shown to be quite useful in a variety of biomedical applications. Naturally produced polymers of protein or carbohydrate origin have also been employed as scaffolds in tissue engineering for many years. Collagen has been the most widely researched natural polymer for scaffold creation. Besides, aliphatic synthetic polymers such as polylactic acid, polyglycolic acid, and polycaprolactone are effective for scaffold fabrication. The improvements in material science have led to the procurement of biomaterials from natural sources, then processed using a variety of techniques, including porogen leaching, gas foaming, phase separation, fiber meshing, and three-dimensional printing. This generates a variety of three-dimensional scaffolds with various porosities and surface characteristics. When compared to the original components, hydroxyapatite composites have been proven to have superior characteristics. In the field of bone tissue repair and engineering, the biological performance of composites containing hydroxyapatite and other abundant natural biopolymers such as chitosan, collagen, gelatin, and cellulose is thoroughly investigated. This chapter discusses the various hydroxyapatite composite scaffolds utilized in *in vitro* and *in vivo* bone tissue engineering investigations, including their fabrication techniques.

Keywords: biomaterials, hydroxyapatite, composite scaffolds, tissue engineering, three-dimensional printing

1. Introduction

Bone deformities frequently demand surgical therapy along with bone grafts. Autografts provide considerable osteogenic properties and are considered as "gold standard." However, donor site morbidity and hematoma have been linked to this procedure. Furthermore, with the limited supply of autografts and the risks associated with allografts, surgeons, and engineers are looking at novel ways to treat bone deformities. Among all the reported methods, tissue engineering is a multidisciplinary approach that integrates biological science and engineering concepts to augment or substitute biological tissues, and it has provided a novel treatment option for bone deformities. Several factors have critical effects on the process of tissue engineering; the scaffolds are one of the key factors, which act as substrate and also provide structural and mechanical support for cell growth. Hydroxyapatite (HA)—one of the main components of natural bone, has widely been applied as scaffolds in tissue engineering owing to its bioactivity and osteoconductivity. Based on these features, HA is an excellent choice for orthopedic and dental implants [1]. Up to now, various HA-based materials (natural and synthetic) have been developed and studied. Nowadays, a variety of materials and manufacturing methods, including 3D printing, is widely regarded as a novel alternative to traditional bone grafts for fabricating sophisticated biological products, such as biological scaffolds, tissues, organs, and customized medical devices, utilizing biological materials, living cells, and signaling molecules, and the use of computer-aided design (CAD) modeling to integrate 3D printing into tissue engineering has substantially improved scaffold production accuracy and repeatability.

In this review, we aim to provide an overview of HA-based materials, their types, and preparation as well as their applications in bone tissue engineering will also be introduced. This review may be useful for researchers interested in bone tissue engineering to receive an insight into HA-based materials and then choose the appropriate material depending on their preferences.

2. Natural sources of hydroxyapatite

Chemically formed HA has long been employed for bone tissue engineering, but its low durability and stability have limited its utility in the biomedical field. Because of the disadvantages of chemically and physically manufactured HA, natural biowastes have been used. Researchers have been attempting to find a way to synthesize HA using natural products. Several studies have shown that natural sources, such as corals, fish scales, eggshells, fish bones, seaweed, and animal bones, can be used for the successful preparation of HA [2]. Organic food waste, such as bovine/fish bones, seashells, and eggshells, may have ideal potential for generating HA, with extremely high availability, which could improve orthopedic applications. Scaffolds can also be made by successfully integrating biodegradable polymers (for adaptive degradation and biocompatibility) and bioceramics (for strength and bioactivity) to improve the bioactivity of the produced materials. With simple and efficient methods, numerous researchers have demonstrated the potential of transforming food waste into immensely useful bioceramics. Animal bones, eggshells, fish bones, oyster shells, and corals have all been used in various synthesis procedures. Additionally, Rocha et al. demonstrated the hydrothermal conversion of natural aragonite from cuttlefish bone in HA. HA derived from biological sources retains many of the attributes of the precursor materials, including chemical composition and pore structure. In this regard, it contains high calcium content as well as important trace minerals for bone formation, such as Mg and Na. The use of biowaste is cost-effective and environmentally friendly. Biowaste, such as eggshells, animal bones, and sea shells, has also shown considerable promise in this direction. The ability to make HA from fish bones has been established in recent years by simple calcination. This method produces HA with a structure and shape that is highly comparable to human bone. Furthermore, all microorganisms and organic components from the source are eliminated by heating it to a high temperature. Furthermore, HA derived from natural sources commonly contains ions such as Mg2+, Na+, Zn2+, and K+. These ions improve the effectiveness of natural HA by encouraging bone growth and regeneration [3].

3. Fabrication techniques for hydroxyapatite-based composite scaffolds

To create scaffolds with the desired properties, HA-based composites have been used in combination with other biomaterials, such as polymers or other inorganic materials. In addition to the "biological" advantages of using such biomaterials, these decrease the requirement for synthetics (materials derived from fossil fuels) in the biomedical business, improving ecological impacts all around.

According to the literature, a variety of techniques can be used to manufacture HA-based composites. Biomimetic mineralization, electrochemical deposition, lyophilization, electrospinning, self-assembling, and chemical vapor deposition are a few of these methods [4].

3.1 3D printing technologies for HA-based nanocomposites

With or without encapsulating cells, the 3D printing process involves the precise layering of biomaterials. The preparation phase, printing phase, and post-handling phase make up the majority of the entire process. In the preliminary stage, computer graphics tools, such as CAD/CAM and biomaterials, are used. *In vitro* transplantation, animal implantation, and tissue maturation in bioreactors all include the post-handling procedure. The most popular 3D printing techniques are inkjet printing, stereolithography (SLA), extrusion printing, and laser printing (**Figure 1**) [5].

3.1.1 Inkjet-based 3D printing

Inkjet-based 3D printing with additional names such as drop-on-demand inkjet printing and continuous inkjet uses a nozzle driven by thermal or acoustic forces to eject liquid droplets onto the substrate. Different inkjet printers generate different droplets.

Two distinct methods of inkjet-based 3D printing exist continuous inkjet printing which creates an ongoing stream of liquid drops and drop-on-demand inkjet printing where individual drops are generated. Thermal and piezoelectric drop-on-demand inkjet printing technologies are employed in the drop-on-demand inkjet printing process to create pressure pulses and enhance droplet production and ejection. A small thin-film heater is used in the fluid chamber of the thermal drop-on-demand inkjet printing technique so that the fluid in direct contact with the heater can be heated more easily by applying a voltage gradient across the heater. Small vapor pockets or bubbles can form more easily when the fluid is heated continuously above its boiling point. Since there is no longer any heat transmission from the heater to the fluid, these bubbles quickly deflate when there is no voltage gradient. Using mechanical actuation, the piezoelectric drop-on-demand inkjet printing technique creates a pressure pulse. The liquid phase is used during the inkjet-based 3D printing process in both of the approaches [6].

Strobel et al. [7] generated the porous biphasic calcium phosphate (BCP) scaffolds *via* indirect 3D printing of a powder composed of homogenized 35 wt.% HA,

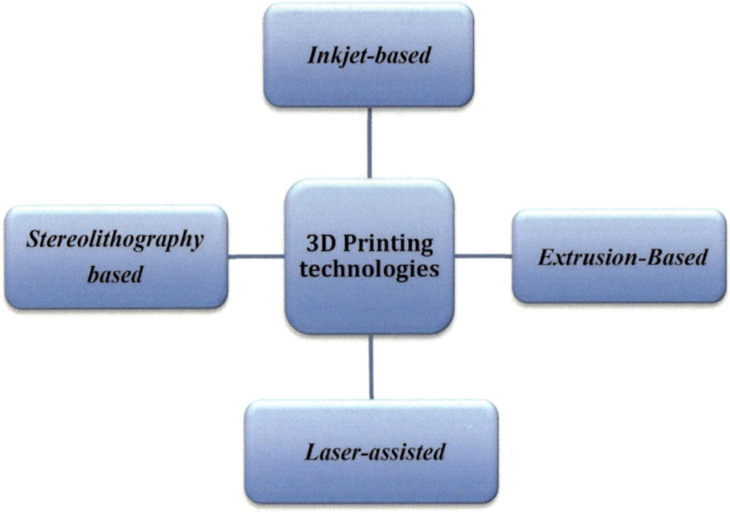

Figure 1.
Most popular 3D printing techniques.

35 wt.% TCP, and 30 wt.% of a modified potato starch powder. Starch consolidation led to considerable porosity. Additionally, growth factor (BMP-2) and osteogenic cells (primary osteoblasts) were seeded and cultured for a few weeks in a flow bioreactor. Warnke et al. also printed BCP scaffolds by 3D printing, and the BCP scaffold was seeded with human osteoblasts [7].

3.1.2 Stereolithography (SLA)-based 3D printing

The "father of 3D printing," Chuck Hull, invented SLA, which is typically used to create polymeric constructs. SLA, where a platform moves the scaffold after each new layer is built while a photoreactive resin is selectively cured. An ultraviolet (UV) laser beam is employed in the SLA-based 3D printing method to selectively cure the photopolymer resin. SLA-based 3D printing provides many benefits over inkjet-based printing, including fast speed, high resolution, and consistency. This technique employs a digital mirror array, usually, either UV light or near-UV blue light (405 nm) is employed.

Woesz et al., utilizing visible light, showed the use of printing systems. They fabricated microporous HA scaffolds using the SLA approach with visible light; the scaffold had a strut size of 450 m, with designed, fully interconnected macro-porosity. Although the SLA approach has been used for 3D printing, Le Guéhennec et al. claimed that the use of SLA for 3D printing of HA composites is constrained by several issues. For instance, the entrapment of unreacted monomers and residuals and the use of photoinitiators and radicals may compromise the integrity of the bone matrix synthesis in addition to elevating the risk of cytotoxicity. Despite these challenges, the incorporation of HA *via* SLA has the overall effect of promoting bone regeneration due to the increase in osteoblast activity on the HA surface [8, 9].

3.1.3 Extrusion-based 3D printing

The principle of extrusion-based 3D printing relies on extruding a viscous material using an extruder that is steered through a mechanical or electromagnetic actuator to create 3D objects According to Derakhshanfar et al., the extrusion-based 3D printing technique is characterized by different extrusion systems that can be cataloged as pneumatic pressure, piston, and screw-driven systems. Numerous benefits are available for extrusion-based 3D printing, including high cell seeding density, rapid printing, and scalability. The printed structures may then be cross-linked utilizing ionic, photo, and thermal crosslinking methods. This printing technology can also be utilized to manufacture continuous cylindrical filaments using various types of inks.

Direct ink writing (DIW, also known as robocasting) and fused deposition modeling (FDM), in which the raw material is expelled by a nozzle, are the two extrusion-based methods. The process of FDM is based on heating the material (polymer and polymer-ceramic composites) before squeezing it out of a nozzle, and by moving the nozzle, the material is deposited on a substrate, layer-by-layer.

The resulting printed constructs are subsequently heat treated to eliminate the binder and densify the ceramic. Sun et al. also utilized the DIW technique in applying silk fibroin ink, filled with HA nanoparticles, to print 3D scaffolds characterized by gradient pore spacings, ranging from 200 to 750 nm through the DIW technique [10, 11].

3.1.4 Laser-assisted 3D printing

The working principle relies on a pulsed laser beam for deposition of bio-ink, including cells, onto a substrate to fabricate 3D objects. The component of the printing system includes a pulsed laser source, a target coated with the substance to be printed (also known as ribbon), and a receiving substrate. Deckard and Beaman created printing in 1986 at the University of Texas in Austin in the United States. A powerful laser beam is focused onto the powder bed during SLS printing to selectively and continuously irradiate the surface of the powders, fusing them to produce the 3D construct. Xia et al. fabricated nano-HA/poly-caprolactone (PCL), using the SLS technology, such that the porosity (78.54–70.31%) and mechanical strength (1.38–3.17 MPa) of the printed scaffold could be regulated by variation of the printing parameters. The printed nano-HA/PCL scaffolds were more bioactive than the PCL scaffolds, according to the *in vitro* data. Compared to HA, BCP is usually challenging to fabricate as a porous scaffold by SLS printing because of the short sintering time. The sintering ability of BCP ceramics can be significantly improved *via* compositing with polymers [12].

3.2 Hydroxyapatite (HA) and HA-based nanocomposites *via* 3D printing

3.2.1 Hydroxyapatite

The hexagonal crystalline structure of hydroxyapatite (HA), also known as $Ca_{10}(PO_4)_6(OH)_2$, is what distinguishes it from other minerals and is what gives bone its mineralized components. Additionally, HA possesses good physicochemical qualities, such as osteoconductivity, bioactivity, resorbability, and delayed decomposition characteristics. Furthermore, nanometer-sized HA can increase intracellular absorption and lower cell survival *in vitro*.

Due to the lack of bonding and flowability for the printing process, considerable study on pure-HA printed materials has not been done, despite the fact that HA is widely considered for hard tissue regeneration due to its presence in the native extracellular matrix (ECM) of bone tissue. To print precise HA structures, various kinds of sacrificial materials and polymers are used as binders during the 3D printing process [13].

3.2.2 Hydroxyapatite (HA)/polymer-based nanocomposites

The printability of HA constructions can be improved by combining a polymer with HA nanoparticles. Due to the suitability and compatibility with cellular environments, various polymers could be used to fabricate (no matter how complex) constructs in ambient or relatively mild chemical and environmental conditions (**Table 1**) [14].

3.2.2.1 HA/collagen nanocomposites

Collagen, fibrin, gelatin, silk, and other high-weight biomacromolecules found in nature can be employed as bio-ink network precursors. The amino acid sequences in natural polymers, such as collagen and gelatin, specifically the adhesion ligand arginine-glycine-aspartic acid (RGD), make them ideal for cell attachment. Collagen refers to a family of fibrillary proteins with a triple-helix structure of polyproline-II (PP-II) type. Significantly, collagen type I represents 90% of the collagen present in the human body, mainly in the skin, bones, tendons, and organs. The main structural element of the ECM is type I collagen, which is also frequently employed as a 3D hydrogel. Collagen/HA (collagen type I) was created by Lin et al. using a low-temperature robocasting technique. The 3D structure of the printed scaffolds was remarkable. *In vivo* data show that the printed scaffolds with interconnected pores might facilitate cell penetration and mineralization and further enhance bone regeneration after being implanted in a rabbit femoral condyle lesion model. A homogenous collagen/HA suspension was generated by Montalbano et al. using rod-like HA nanoparticles combined with type I collagen and an ammonium-based dispersion agent (Darvan 821-A). This suspension was used as bio-ink for extrusion 3D printing. The obtained collagen/HA bio-ink showed that the shear thinning and sol-gel transition upon stimulus-physiological conditions and the mesh-like constructs could be printed [15].

Hydroxyapatite-based nanocomposites
HA/collagen nanocomposites
Hydroxyapatite (HA)/gelatin nanocomposites
Hydroxyapatite (HA)/silk nanocomposites
Hydroxyapatite (HA)/alginate nanocomposites
Hydroxyapatite (HA)/cellulose nanocomposites
Hydroxyapatite (HA)/chitosan nanocomposites
Hydroxyapatite (HA)/poly (lactic acid)-based nanocomposites
Hydroxyapatite (HA)/poly-caprolactone nanocomposites
Hydroxyapatite (HA)/polymethyl methacrylate nanocomposites
Hydroxyapatite (HA)/polyvinyl alcohol nanocomposites
Hydroxyapatite (HA)/poly (propylene fumarate) nanocomposites

Table 1.
Hydroxyapatite-based nanocomposites.

3.2.2.2 Hydroxyapatite (HA)/gelatin nanocomposites

Compared to collagen, gelatine presents no cytotoxicity, good cell adhesion, faster biodegradability, easier preparation, and low cost, thus it can be considered as a sufficient candidate for printing.

Animal tissues from diverse species, including those from pigs, cows, and fish, can be used to create gelatin polymers with a range of molecular weights and isoelectric points. The combined use of gelatine and loaded HA presents an ideal microenvironment for cell adhesion, proliferation, and differentiation toward an osteogenic phenotype, due to the presence of intrinsically cell adhesive motifs of gelatin. The combined use of gelatin and HA was demonstrated in the study by Samadikuchaksaraei et al. [15] where an HA/gelatin scaffold was fabricated using the layer solvent casting in combination with lamination techniques. The prepared HA/gelatin scaffold could support osteoblasts' adhesion and growth, and *in vivo* results confirm that the scaffold could accelerate collagen content during bone healing. Nosrati et al. fabricated a HA/gelatin scaffold using a 3D printing method, with reduced graphene oxide (rGO) nanosheets used to reinforce the printed scaffold. The addition of rGO/HA could result in smaller pores and higher 3D accuracy of scaffolds. Notably, the gelatin may also be applied in drug release, due to its induction of degradation and deposition on the apatite layer [16, 17].

3.2.2.3 Hydroxyapatite (HA)/silk nanocomposites

Silk fibroin (SF), a protein fiber generated from Bombyx mori cocoons, has traditionally been employed as a natural polymer in the production of surgical sutures. Due to its unique structure, which consists of hydrophobic sheet crystalline blocks staggered by hydrophilic amorphous acidic spacers, SF possesses outstanding mechanical properties and good biocompatibility both *in vitro* and *in vivo* [18].

SF has also established a good reputation for bone TE applications due to its many unique properties, including impressive biocompatibility, strong mechanical behavior, minimal/non-immunogenicity, biodegradability, and ease of processability. Furthermore, the silk fibroin scaffolds showed improved anticoagulant activity. According to Lee JW et al. [19], HA/SF composites can encourage bone repair by activating signaling pathways linked to cell-biomaterial interactions. The obtained 3D printed scaffolds showed good porosity of 70% with interconnected pores with a diameter of ~400 m and relatively high compressive strength of over 6 MPa. While retaining cell adhesion and penetration, the printed scaffolds also showed well *in vitro* biomineralization activity in SBF.

3.2.2.4 Hydroxyapatite (HA)/alginate nanocomposites

The alginate structure is composed of a linear repetition of (1,4)-linked-D-mannuronic acid (M) and L-guluronic acid (G) units, with 4C1 ring conformation. Alginate has a strong affinity for di- and tri-valent cations and rapidly forms a gel in the presence of low concentrations of such ions (Mg2+ being an exception) at a range of pH values and temperatures. Alginate is also a polysaccharide that is negatively charged and works well as a scaffold for cell growth. Alginate can be modified by adding functional groups (such as heparin) that can bind to and immobilize various growth factors. These changes allow the growth factors to be micropatterned in three dimensions. Several studies have also indicated that HA/alginate nanocomposites are suitable for TE, with enhanced bioactivity [20].

Pre-crosslinking the HA/alginate nanocomposite with D-gluconic acid lactone improved the mechanical characteristics of the printed HA/alginate scaffold (GDL). To ensure continuous drug release, curcumin, an anti-inflammatory medicine, might be added to the printed scaffold during printing. According to *in vitro* experiments, the mouse bone mesenchymal stem cells (mBMSCs) may have adhered to the porous HA/alginate scaffolds. Curcumin, an anti-inflammatory medication, could be placed onto the printed scaffold during printing to achieve sustained drug release. The mouse bone mesenchymal stem cells (mBMSCs) may have attached to the porous HA/alginate scaffolds, according to *in vitro* studies [21].

3.2.2.5 Hydroxyapatite (HA)/cellulose nanocomposites

The most prevalent naturally occurring polymeric material in nature is cellulose, which is a well-known fact. Cellulose is used in TE because of its great biocompatibility, particular protein-binding locations, and remarkable mechanical strength. The high density of reactive hydroxyl groups on cellulose fiber can also aid in the immobilization of cell adhesion proteins like fibronectin on the surface of cellulose. Biocompatible cellulose fiber can be used to create a variety of scaffolds. Liu H et al. [22] fabricated HA/bacterial cellulose nanocomposites by inkjet 3D printing, which could be applied in bone engineering. Favi et al. [23] prepared HA/bacterial cellulose scaffold with well-defined honeycomb pore arrays using a laser patterning technique. The fabricated scaffold was shown to have a honeycomb pore array with a diameter of 300 m, which was suitable for bone TE applications. The nanocomposite scaffold can have good mechanical strength because of the addition of HA to cellulose. The nanocomposite scaffold can have good mechanical strength because of the addition of HA to cellulose. However, more research is required to determine whether HA/cellulose bio-ink can be printed in 3D.

3.2.2.6 Hydroxyapatite (HA)/chitosan nanocomposites

Chitin is converted into the polysaccharide complex chitosan, which has strong biocompatibility, degradability, and solubility in weak acids, and is nontoxic. Chitosan is a linear copolymer of -(1–4) linked 2-acetamido-2-deoxy-Dglucopyranose and 2-amino-2-deoxy-D-glucopyranose. Being a positively charged polysaccharide, chitosan still needs to be chemically altered and/or combined with other biomaterials to achieve the best mechanical and physiological qualities for TE. There are several reports on HA-reinforced chitosan scaffolds fabricated using different methods, including 3D printing. The high uniformity of the structure enhanced the mechanical strength of the printed HA/chitosan scaffold, thus improving its capacity to maintain its shape during the shrinkage phase of the dispensing medium.

Venkatesan J et al. [24] discovered that the mechanical property of HA/chitosan composites could be regulated by adjusting the weight ratio of HA/chitosan, such that the maximum value of the compressive strength attains 120 MPa at a mass ratio of HA/chitosan of 70/30. The printed HA/chitosan nanocomposites scaffold offers a wide range of possible applications in bone TE because of these great features.

3.2.2.7 Hydroxyapatite (HA)/poly-(lactic acid) based nanocomposites

Poly (lactic acid), sometimes known as PLA, is a nontoxic, biodegradable thermoplastic polymer created by the ring-open polymerization of lactide. Sugar feedstock fermentation is a source of PLA. Because of its linear aliphatic structure, PLA has appealing biodegradability, outstanding biocompatibility, and great mechanical qualities. For the above reasons, PLA was widely used as a matrix material in constructing biodegradable composites for bone repair, and bone fixation devices used in orthopedics and oral surgery applications. However, due to its unpredictable hydrolysis and weak hydrophilicity, PLA still has a narrow range of applications. However, these issues might be resolved by fusing PLA and bioactive ceramics like HA.

In the beginning, the HA/PLA composite was thought of as a viable biomaterial for bone replacement and repair. The distribution of HA nanoparticles may delay the rate at which PLA degrades, while increasing the distribution of HA nanoparticles may enhance mechanical properties. By using finite element modeling and simulation, the compression strength of printed structures could be changed. The authors claim that printed HA/PLA scaffold exhibited a greater rate of cell adhesion and proliferation than PLA scaffold based on *in vitro* studies. Using FDM, Domenech M et al. [25] created HA microspheres/PLA scaffold. HA/PLA scaffolds displayed increased porosity and a rougher surface compared to printed PLA scaffolds. Poly-L-lactic acid (PLLA) degrades more slowly than PLA, which is thought to lead to a slower inflammatory tissue reaction. Due to the bioresorbable characteristic, HA/PLLA has bone-bonding potential for bone regeneration [25].

3.2.2.8 Hydroxyapatite (HA)/poly-caprolactone nanocomposites

Poly-caprolactone (PCL) is commonly used as a synthetic biomaterial for bone tissue and periodontal applications due to its biocompatibility, suitability for various scaffold fabrication techniques, prolonged degradation rate, and mechanical stability. However, due to PCL's slow rate of disintegration and prolonged durations of intactness, scaffolds may have a negative impact on bone repair. Because PCL and PCL-based scaffolds are easily printable and quickly solidify following extrusion, they can be produced using 3D printing. PCL and PCL-based scaffolds could be easily fabricated *via* 3D printing because of their good printability, and quick solidification after extrusion. Yang Hu et al. [26] fabricated HA/PCL scaffolds with hierarchical porous structures and tunable multifunctional performance *via* 3D printing. Peter SJ et al. [27] also fabricated HA/PCL scaffolds using the SLS technique. The printed scaffolds had porosity ranging from 78.54 to 70.31%, and the corresponding compressive strength ranged from 1.38 to 3.17 MPa. The *in vivo* results confirm that the printed HA/PCL scaffolds not only enhanced the formation of new bone but also orthopedic and reconstructive surgery. Xia et al. also fabricated HA/PCL scaffolds using the SLS technique. The printed scaffolds had porosity ranging from 78.54 to 70.31%, and the corresponding compressive strength ranged from 1.38 to 3.17 MPa. The *in vivo* outcomes demonstrate that the printed HA/PCL scaffolds not only improved new bone development but also satiated all the fundamental criteria for bone TE scaffolds, indicating a sizable potential for usage in orthopedic and reconstructive surgery.

3.2.2.9 Hydroxyapatite (HA)/polymethyl methacrylate nanocomposites

Polymethyl methacrylate (PMMA) is an FDA-approved synthetic polymer widely employed in ophthalmic, orthopedic, and dental applications. PMMA is also used as bone cement to fill defects of any shape or size, As a result, it can be used to treat osseous malignancies, trauma, illnesses, and birth defects in the skeletal structure. Lal B et al. [28] developed HA/PMMA using solvent casting particulate leaching technique;

computational fluid dynamics (CFD) analysis concluded that HA/PMMA scaffold with 60 wt.% HA content tended to be the most potential option for bone TE applications due to the finest compromise between porosity, permeability, and compressive strength.

As filaments for 3D printing, Esmi et al. combined HA/PMMA with carbon nanotubes (CNTs). The modulus and hardness of HA/PMMA/CNTs were found to be greater than those of HA/PMMA using nano-indentation, and the generated nanocomposites accelerated cell adhesion, growth, and proliferation, according to the findings of a biocompatibility test [29].

3.2.2.10 Hydroxyapatite (HA)/polyvinyl alcohol nanocomposites

PVA, a thermoplastic that dissolves in water, is frequently utilized as a support material in 3D printing. Due to its excellent biocompatibility, high water solubility, and chemical resistance, it is often used in medical equipment. PVA is mostly used in cartilage TE because it has a tensile strength that is comparable to that of human articular cartilage. Notably, compositing PVA with calcium phosphate nanoparticles, such as HA, TCP, and BCP, showed promising applications for the fabrication of scaffolds in bone TE. The osteoconductive HA/PVA scaffold could be created for bone replacement, according to several research findings. For instance, Nie L et al. [30] fabricated HA/PVA scaffolds by powder-based 3D printing. The results show that the printed scaffold with 1.0 wt.% of PVA showed the best compressive strength. The HA/PVA scaffolds' performances were superior and considerably more appropriate as bone scaffolds than those of the HA/polyvinylpyrrolidone (PVP) and HA/polyacrylamide (PAM) scaffolds made using the same method. In addition, the printed HA/PVA produced had good cytocompatibility.

3.2.2.11 Hydroxyapatite (HA)/poly (propylene fumarate) nanocomposites

Unsaturated linear polyester poly (propylene fumarate, or PPF), which has carbon double bonds throughout its backbone, can be crosslinked. PLA, PCL, and PPF are regarded as bioresorbable polymers that can break down *in vivo* either through hydrolysis or through enzymatic cleavage. PPF may be degraded into nontoxic products of propylene glycol, poly (acrylic acid-coumaric acid), and fumaric acid. Numerous medical applications, including vascular stents, cartilage, blood vessel engineering, bone TE, have made significant use of PRF. This may be printed into a variety of 3D shapes using extrusion-based printing and SLA3D printing. Besides linear PPF oligomers, Fer et al. [31] developed PPF bio-ink for continuous DLP, with the printing speed improved. PPF is one of the promising candidate materials for load-bearing applications due to its suitable mechanical properties. But PPF still needs to have its biomechanical and osteoconductive qualities improved, perhaps by adding ceramic components. Lee et al. [32] asserted that the osteoconductive ability of HA/PPF nanocomposites was increased compared with pure PPF. Lee et al. fabricated HA/PPF scaffolds with micro-SLA (MSTL) technology. During the preparation of the HA/PPF bio-ink, diethyl fumarate (DEF) was incorporated to reduce the viscosity, and the photo-initiator bis-acyl phosphine oxide (BAPO) and 7 wt.% of HA were designed. Interconnected pores could be seen in the printed scaffolds. Additionally, *in vitro* research indicates that printed HA/PPF scaffolds promoted MC3T3-E1 cells' proliferation and cell adhesion more effectively than PPF scaffolds did.

3.3 Hydroxyapatite (HA)-based ceramics

3.3.1 Hydroxyapatite (HA)/beta-tricalcium phosphate (BCP)-based ceramics

Beta-tricalcium phosphate is of low mechanical strength and degrades too quickly in a physiological environment which can be improved *via* its combination with HA. For 30 years, BCP has been utilized to create bone graft materials; BCP-based ceramics have demonstrated clinical success. Asran AS [33] fabricated porous BCP ceramics using extrusion-based 3D printing with a motor-assisted micro-syringe (MAM) system; the morphology, pore size, and porosity of printed BCP scaffolds could be precisely controlled to optimize their mechanical properties.

3.3.2 Hydroxyapatite (HA)/bioglass-based ceramics

The field of bioactive inorganic materials, which may bind with bone tissues, was introduced by the discovery of bioglass. Due to its osteoconductivity and osteoproductivity, bioglass has demonstrated significant potential in bone regeneration. According to numerous investigations, the remarkable bioactivity of HA/bioglass composites makes them suitable for use in bone regeneration. However, bioglass scaffolds may deteriorate before the formation of new bone due to the rapid rate of bioglass dissolution in bodily fluids. Ferraz MP et al. [34] indicated that HA/bioglass could stimulate early osteogenesis and osteointegration at the interface in the biological environment. For instance, Zebarjad SM et al. [35] fabricated the calcium sulfate hydrate (CSH)/mesoporous bioactive glass (MBG) scaffolds using the inkjet 3D printing approach (4th 3D Bioplotter™, EnvisionTEC GmbH, Germany). The printed scaffolds were well used for apatite mineralization because of their regular and consistent structure. Seyedmajidi et al. additionally acquired HA/bioactive glass for use as cell scaffolds in the restoration of the rat tibia. The radiographic, histological, and histomorphometric evaluations showed that the trabecular thickness and rate of new bone formation were elevated.

3.3.3 HA-based composites of titanium ceramics

Besides calcium phosphate ceramics, titanium and its alloys, such as titanium dioxide (TiO_2) and titanium alloy (Ti-6Al-4 V, Ti64), can be used to fabricate scaffolds for TE. TiO_2 is also capable of enhancing the growth of bone and vascular tissues and osteoconductivity. For instance, Kim et al. created HA/TiO_2 nanocomposites utilizing HA-doped TiO_2 particles and concluded that these materials had greater strength and bioactivity than TiO_2 compounds. Additionally, Ti64, known for its excellent strength-to-weight ratio, is an alloy that can be employed in fabricating porous scaffolds. SLM, or selective laser melting, can be used to create such porous Ti64 scaffolds.

However, since Ti64 lacks some functionality, such as blood compatibility and bone conductivity, the surface of Ti64 may be coated using HA to improve its physicochemical properties as demonstrated in the literature. For instance, Cai X et al. [36] used a nanorod-structured HA as a coating on the surface of Ti64 *via* atmospheric plasma spraying in combination with hydrothermal treatment and subsequently demonstrated how the created nano-structured surface will improve osseointegration and cell responses.

4. Different types of hydroxyapatite polymer composite for bone tissue engineering

4.1 Hydroxyapatite as tissue scaffolding material

Hydroxyapatite (HA) ($Ca_{10}(PO_4)_6(OH)_2$) is a biocompatible ceramic material that belongs to the calcium phosphate cement family (CPCs). Natural bones are mainly made up of HA, collagen, and water. Biological apatite, the main mineral form present in mammals is a carbonate-rich, hydroxyl-deficient apatite with a Ca/P ratio of less than 1.67. Synthetic HA has a comparable composition and characteristics to natural HA found in bones and teeth. Synthetic HA is also a biocompatible, bioactive, nontoxic, and osteoinductive substance. In two alternative scaffold material combinations, HA can be utilized. Hydroxyapatite has significant remodeling and cell adhesive qualities when combined with natural materials, but it can also trigger an immunological response. Gelatin, fibrinogen, and collagen are examples of natural materials (**Figure 2**). Synthetic materials, on the other hand, are less likely to elicit an immune response, although they can still be hazardous [37].

4.2 Hydroxyapatite in combination with natural materials

4.2.1 Collagen

Collagen is a natural substance that is biodegradable, porous, and biocompatible. It is a natural component of many soft and hard tissues and provides raw protein for the ECM. They are made up of 28 different proteins that fall into six different categories:

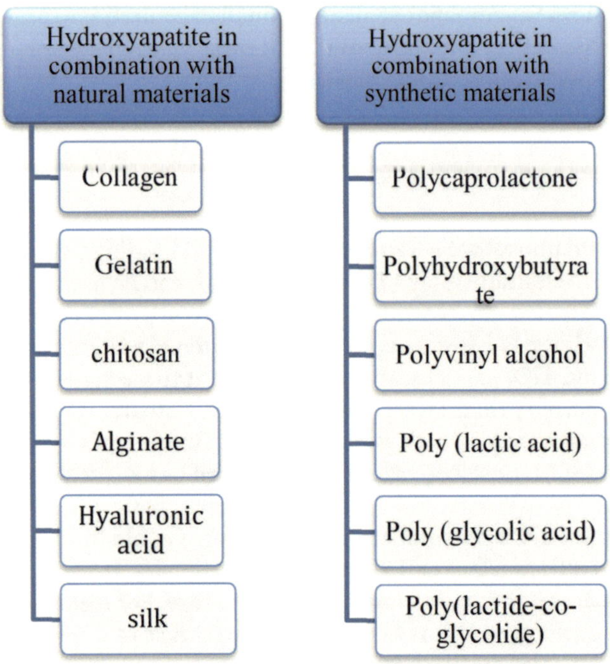

Figure 2.
Natural and synthetic materials used in combination with hydroxyapatite.

fibrillar, fibril-associated collagens with interrupted triple helices (FACIT), beaded filament, basement membrane, short-chain, and transmembrane collagens. Because type I collagen is plentiful in the bones, it is the molecule of interest when it comes to bone regeneration. Collagen, on the other hand, lacks stiffness, making its usage in load-bearing regions challenging [37].

The idea of creating collagen (Col)-HA biocomposites is supported since they make up the microarchitecture of the bones. Collagen has long been known for its high biocompatibility, low degradation, and positive interactions with cells and other organic macromolecules in our bodies. To stimulate osteogenic differentiation—HA biocomposites combine collagen's cell migration and binding capabilities with HA's inherent bioactivity. Collagen improves the mechanical strength of porous HA scaffolds by reducing porosity. The increased mechanical strength is due to the creation of intermolecular H-bonds between collagen and HA, which raises fracture energy and hence improves failure resistance. Because of all these factors, tissue engineering can also be done with collagen-HA composites. When implanted in the rat tibia, these scaffolds exhibited osteoconductivity and begin to disintegrate after 12 weeks. In animal tests, these collagen-HA composite materials have also been employed to cover titanium implants with encouraging results. Collagen-HA scaffolds containing recombinant growth factors and antibiotics are also being developed which helps to improve regeneration [37]. Hoyer et al. created resorbable collagen/hydroxyapatite porous scaffolds with appropriate connectivity and mechanical characteristics (2012) [38]. Sotome et al. further verified the advantages of porous HAp-collagen composite for bone regeneration. Collagen-Hap was also successfully used for cheekbone augmentation, resulting in significant ossification with little inflammation and limiting bone development over time.

4.2.2 Gelatin

Gelatin is a natural polymer made from collagen that has been denatured. It's been employed in adipose tissue, blood vessels, bone, intervertebral disc, muscle, tendon, heart, liver, and skin tissue engineering. Bone tissue engineering can also be facilitated by gelatin/HA scaffolds. In terms of osteogenic development of periodontal ligament cells, these scaffolds have demonstrated encouraging outcomes. Due to the immunogenic reaction induced by collagen by-products, an alternative organic matrix component source was necessary as a backup. In this case, the organic component in the composite was preferable to gelatin. The role of gelatin as a matrix was investigated after it was degraded in lysozyme under physiological circumstances. In thermal solution, gelatin is a linear, amorphous, hydrophilic, and moldable biomaterial and also biocompatible, and has a slower rate of degradation, and the by-products are not immunogenic. The addition of gum to the HA/gelatin composite can improve the mechanical characteristics of the scaffold. The scaffolds are seeded with Mesenchymal Stem Cells (MSCs) extracted from Wharton jelly that protects the umbilical cord. According to White et al., the preparation of gelatin-HAp composite can be done through the casting method as it is a simple and economical approach in the preparation of porous scaffold materials [39].

Because of their biodegradability and biocompatibility, gelatin and hydroxyapatite films in various ratios appear to have promise in bone tissue engineering, according to the findings of multiple research. However, in order to accurately assess the mechanical characteristics of this composite, additional detailed experiments were necessary.

4.2.3 Chitosan

Chitosan (CS) is a D-glucosamine/N-acetyl-D-glucosamine copolymer, which is a versatile natural biopolymer made by partial deacetylation of chitin under alkaline environments. Chitin and its derivatives have received a lot of interest as a scaffold material in bone tissue engineering. Pure chitosan scaffolds, on the other hand, have poor mechanical characteristics and lack osteoconductivity. HA can be employed to improve the ability of CS to differentiate into osteoblasts [40]. By including HA in the CS scaffolds, the bioactivity and biocompatibility of the CS can be improved. CS/HA systems have also been employed as carriers to transport drugs, stem cells, and other growth factors into hosts. The very first attempt to create a CS/HA biocomposite material was the creation of a bone-filling cement made of powdered HA/ZnO/CaO combined in a chitosan sol. The final paste had a quick setting time and a high compressive strength. The HA nanoparticles are evenly distributed throughout the CS matrix, and the HA crystallites increase during nucleation due to interactions generated between calcium ions and CS amino acids [40]. The aggregation of HA nanoparticles is a disadvantage of this type of material; however, Hu et al. devised a simple *in situ* hybridization approach to make HA/CS nanocomposites that can overcome this issue. Furthermore, the biocompatibility of the HA/CS scaffold is quite excellent.

The HA/CS composite improved cell adherence, spreading, and proliferation of human mesenchymal stem cells as compared to a pure chitosan scaffold. HA/CS biocomposites have been shown to stimulate bone growth in a variety of bone defects by inducing osteoinduction and osseointegration. To repair the femoral condyle defect in 43 adults New Zealand white rabbits, HA/CS and pure chitosan were implanted into the left femoral condyle. The results demonstrated that after 12 weeks of surgery, rabbits implanted with the HA/CS scaffold had completely healed their bone abnormalities, whereas the defects remained in the pure chitosan group. The HA/CS composite can also be employed as a functional layer on other implants to create outstanding osteoinduction characteristics. Wang et al., for example, coated HA/CS on a titanium surface(cTi) and employed it in diabetic patients. After 12 weeks, the cTi implant had greater bone contact and a higher volume of new bone formed into it than the Ti implants [41].

4.2.4 Alginate

Alginate (Alg) is a marine-sourced biopolymer produced from brown algae, similar to chitosan. Alginates, which produce partially soluble hydrogels in water after partial interaction with divalent cations, have a variety of uses in bone regeneration, wound healing, and drug administration. According to Becker et al., who also researched their mechanical characteristics, alginates are biodegradable and biocompatible materials [42]. This study discovered a link between biocompatibility and alginates purity, with pure versions causing less unfavorable reactions in tissues than their less purified equivalents. In comparison with hydrogels with high mannuronic acid concentration, hydrogels with high glucuronic acid content had improved tensile strength and ductility qualities.

Ceramics, such as HA, can be used to strengthen the mechanical qualities of alginate. Some studies also discovered that a slight increase in Sodium Alginate (SA) content resulted in the production of biocomposites with enhanced density and hardness due to decreased porosity and the establishment of strong linkages within the SA, allowing SA/HA composites to outperform pure SA scaffolds mechanically. *In vitro* and *in vivo* tests were performed on biocomposites including carbonated nano-HA with strontium and sodium alginate (SrCHA) spheres and without strontium (CHA). Vancomycin-loaded Alg/Sr-HA microspheres had improved sustained drug release capabilities. Although the mechanical characteristics of Alg/HA composites are sufficient to fill critical-sized defects (tissue defects which are the smallest one and that do not heal on their own over the course of an animal's lifespan), their usefulness for treating defects in long bones requires additional investigation.

4.2.5 Hyaluronic acid

Hyaluronic acid (HylA) is a hydrophilic linear unbranched glycosaminoglycan composed of repeated N-acetyl glucosamine and glucuronic acid disaccharide units. This was first obtained from the vitreous humor of cows. Because of its elasticity, biocompatibility, antibacterial, and osteoinductive qualities, HylA got a variety of biological uses, including bone regeneration. HylA is engaged in cell signaling pathways and contributes to cell proliferation and differentiation. Bakos et al. investigated the effect of HylA on HA. HylA-conjugated HA/Col composites had a more compact structure and higher bend strength than non-conjugated HA/Col composites, indicating that HylA has a positive impact on the mechanical properties of HA/Col scaffolds [43]. Hyaluronic acid (HylA) is a hydrophilic linear carbohydrate that is found in the body. When the ability of biocomposite scaffolds made of calcium sulfate/HA/HylA and encapsulated with collagenase to repair alveolar bone defects in rats was investigated, it was shown that these scaffolds displayed excellent biocompatibility, compressive strength, and a sustained release of the collagenase enzyme for up to 4 days. Histological analysis of the rat models revealed that defects filled with calcium sulfate HA/HylA-collagenase scaffolds showed significant and uniform regeneration of the alveolar bones 8 weeks post-implantation verified by the increased number of osteocytes observed on the defect site. However, in *in vivo* circumstances, fast enzymatic degradation of HylA must be considered, as this might deplete the mechanical characteristics of HylA-based composites [44].

4.2.6 Silk

Silk may be utilized as a scaffold for MSCs since it is biocompatible and strong. To make the silk/HA scaffold, NaCl can be employed as a porogen. Scaffolds with different HA percentages are made and employed with MSCs cells. According to Bhumiratana et al., since HA stimulates mineralization and trabeculae development in its scaffold, silk/HA scaffolds can play an important role in osteogenic cell differentiation [45].

4.3 Hydroxyapatite in combination with synthetic materials

Natural materials are undeniably accessible and biocompatible, but synthetic materials, under their regulated nature, have many distinct features. Polylactic acid (PLA), poly (lactic-co-glycolic acid) (PLGA), b-tricalcium phosphate (b-TCP), and polycaprolactone (PCL) are examples of synthetic materials. It's also possible to employ HA in conjunction with synthetic materials (**Figure 2**).

4.3.1 Polycaprolactone (PCL)

PCL is a biocompatible, synthetic polymer with easily adjustable mechanical characteristics. PCL (in its high molecular weight form) is recognized for its typical slow breakdown rate of up to 3 years to entirely eradicate itself from the host body, despite the fact that it is biodegradable. The volume of HA in the composite affects the mechanical characteristics of PCL/HA scaffolds. Researchers used laser sintering to create nano-HA (nHA)/PCL scaffolds. Increased nHA concentration leads to osteoblast development and mineralization, based on Alizarin Red and ALP staining. The greatest amount of nHA-containing scaffolds exhibits a slow-release profile of recombinant bone morphogenic protein; as a result, HA/PCL scaffolds are crucial in bone tissue regeneration. The utilization of a biphasic calcium phosphate (BCP) scaffold covered with nHA and PCL for the differentiation of primary human osteoblasts (HOBs) and ASCs cells has been described. The addition of HA to porous PCL has an effect on the latter's behavior under *in vitro* circumstances. Shor et al. in an 11–21 days observational study revealed that porous PCL/HA scaffolds cause an increase in cell survival and proliferation of fetal bovine osteoblasts over conventional PCL scaffolds. Throughout the observation period, cell differentiation as evaluated by alkaline phosphatase activity revealed that PCL-HA scaffolds clearly outperformed conventional PCL scaffolds in terms of alkaline phosphatase activity. In comparison with the negative controls, PCL-HA matrices implanted subcutaneously in white rats demonstrated the development of connective tissues after 7 days and vascularization after 14 days, provoking a very low immune response. After 21 days, the matrices commenced to biodegrade, demonstrating their effectiveness and cytocompatibility in *in vivo* animals. PCL, on the other hand, is very hydrophobic, has minimal antibacterial action, and is known to degrade more slowly than poly (L-lactic acid) (PLLA) and poly(glycolic) acid (PGA) [46].

4.3.2 Polyhydroxybutyrate (PHB)

Poly 3-hydroxybutyrate (P3HB) is a crystalline polyester that belongs to the polyhydroxyalkanoates family of polyhydroxyalkanoates produced by bacteria through enzymatic synthesis. Because brittleness is a key disadvantage of P3HB, it is frequently copolymerized with polyhydroxy valerate (PHV) to improve processability. PHB and gelatin can be coupled with nHA to create a bone scaffold that is both osteoconductive and osteoinductive. The nanofibrous scaffold can be employed in conjunction with MSCs to improve bone regeneration potential. In comparison with P3HB control scaffolds, P3HB/nano-HA scaffolds enhance cell proliferation and differentiation of osteoblasts better. Both scaffolds boosted cell survival and proliferation over time, however, the P3HB/nano-HA scaffold had the best outcomes. When tested subcutaneously on rat models, PHB/HA porous scaffolds filled with bone marrow cells showed promise in *in vivo* environments. Forty-five days after implantation, the implants were covered with a thin connective tissue layer. In the pores of the scaffolds, a healthy connective tissue in-growth comprised of matured osteoblasts, macrophages, and capillary was seen, indicating the site of the active bone formation near the implant site, indicating their capacity to support bone regeneration. However, because both P3HB and HA are brittle materials, the mechanical strength of the P3HB/HA biocomposites is a problem. As a result, because of concerns about their long-term mechanical stability, the composite may not be the best option for implant [47].

4.3.3 Polyvinyl alcohol (PVA)

Tissue engineering can be done with polyvinyl alcohol (PVA)/BCP scaffold. Nie et al. created PVA/BCP scaffolds and seeded BMSC cells on them. The biocompatibility of this scaffold was good. The porosity and mechanical characteristics of the scaffolds are similar to those of bone. It improves MSC adherence, making PVA/BCP scaffolds useful in bone tissue engineering [48].

4.3.4 Poly (lactic acid)

Poly (lactic acid) (PLA) is formed when lactic acid undergoes a polyesterification reaction. It exhibits four different forms: poly (L-lactic acid) (PLLA), poly (D-lactic acid) (PDLA), poly (D,L-lactic acid) (PDLLA), and meso-poly(lactic acid). PLA has high tensile strength and Young's modulus in general. These properties, however, range greatly among the various types of PLA, which defines their applicability. PLA/HA biocomposites are employed as scaffolds as well as carriers for delivering medicines and other proteins into the body. The mechanical properties of PLA/HA biocomposites are influenced by the proportion of HA in the composite and the temperature at which it is produced. Calcined PLA/HA composites with around 80% HA had Young's modulus of 10 GPa, which was comparable to the lower limit of a cortical bone, as well as comparable flexural strength and fracture toughness. Increased cell numbers, cell adhesion, expression of bone-specific markers (osteocalcin), and promotion of osteoblast differentiation by alkaline phosphatase activity demonstrate that PLA/HA biocomposites are biocompatible with a wide range of cell lines, including MG-63 osteosarcoma cells, L929 fibroblastic cells, and MC3T3-E1 osteoblastic precursors. In rabbits with bone defects, PLA/nano-HA/collagen scaffolds seeded with rh-BMP2 (recombinant human bone morphogenic protein) exhibited promising signals of bone remodeling. After 8 weeks, the implant showed cellular infiltration into its pores, and after 12 weeks, it had fully integrated into the defect site, demonstrating the formation of new bony (trabecular) tissues and the replacement of the composite, showing the composite's biodegradability and bone regeneration capacity [49].

4.3.5 Poly (glycolic acid)

The semi-crystalline polymer poly (glycolic acid) (PGA) has a high tensile modulus of 12.5 GPa and is insoluble in most organic solvents. PLA and PGA were the first synthetic biodegradable polymers to be approved for use in the fabrication of resorbable sutures by the US Food and Drug Administration. PGA has better mechanical qualities than PLA and degrades faster. In a 1986 study, PGA implants were found to be biocompatible in rabbits with cortical and cancellous bone abnormalities. The implants in the cancellous locations showed the greatest degradation after 12 weeks of implantation, compared to partial degradation in the cortical bones that did not result in an inflammatory response. *In vitro*, PGA/HA composite scaffolds showed excellent resorption and the appropriate porosity for cellular penetration and adhesion. However, due to the stiffness of PGA and the risk of inflammation caused by its breakdown by-products, their biological applications have been limited [50].

4.3.6 Poly (lactide-co-glycolide)

The biocompatibility and mechanical characteristics of PLGA are well known. PLGA is seen as a solution to both PLA and PGA's drawbacks. Researchers were able to solve the problem of premature degradation by copolymerizing the two and altering the homopolymer ratio, which gave them some control over their degradation rates. PLGA having 75% PGA is known to be amorphous and hydrolytically unstable, causing it to degrade more quickly.

PLGA systems are used in areas such as bone, cartilage, and nerve regeneration, in addition to drug delivery. The mechanical characteristics of PLGA are strengthened by HA. Fisher et al. discovered that adding 30 percent nano-HA to PLGA matrices resulted in composites with three times the strength of the polymer alone, as well as a sixfold increase in compressive modulus. The scaffolds were designed to be injectable, and when injected into swine femoral heads, they increased the trabecular bone strength and compressive modulus from 3.5 to 5.9 MPa and 81 to 180 MPa, respectively [51]. In comparison with PLGA control scaffolds, PLGA/nano-HA scaffolds cultivated with mesenchymal stem cells demonstrated larger cell counts, improved cell adherence, increased cell proliferation, and better alkaline phosphatase activity. Twenty-one days after implantation, PLGA/HA scaffolds implanted into rabbit mandibular defects showed the presence of bone trabeculae without any ongoing osteoblast activity, whereas PLGA control scaffolds had a high number of osteoblasts on their surface, indicating increased cellular activity to generate more bone trabeculae. Also, at the end of 6 weeks, the PLGA/HA scaffolds tested positive for the bone markers osteonectin and osteopontin, indicating increasing bone deposition *in vivo* [52].

5. Application in tissue engineering

Tissue engineering with hydroxyapatite (HA) holds a lot of promise. Furthermore, according to current research, 3D printed HA-based nanocomposites serve as 3D templates for cells to attach, proliferate, and maintain their differentiated function in tissue regeneration. Bone, cartilage, applications in dentistry, skin, and drug delivery are just a few of the possibilities for HA-based structures. These applications are briefly covered below (**Figure 3**).

5.1 Bone

Due to the chemical resemblance of calcium phosphates to bone minerals, notably HA ($Ca10(PO4)6(OH)2$), bioceramic materials are used in bone replacement applications. In comparison with autografts and allografts, a complex hierarchical artificially engineered bone scaffold with a complex structure can reduce the risk of infection, immune response, and transmission of the disease. The optimally designed bond scaffold should meet a number of requirements, including biocompatibility, osteoconduction, osteoinduction, and mechanical properties. In conjunction with natural and synthetic polymers, pure HA or other ceramics such as tetra calcium phosphate can be utilized to build scaffolds for hard tissue regeneration. Polymers, by their very nature, are flexible and lack stiffness. When inorganic materials and polymers are mixed, composite materials display both inorganic features like mechanical strength and flexibility, as well as polymer properties such as porosity and osteoconductivity.

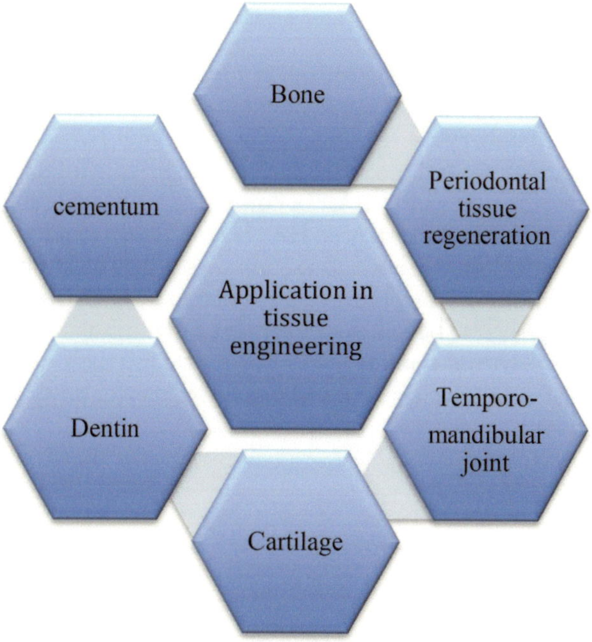

Figure 3.
Applications in tissue engineering.

PLGA/HA is a biocompatible and osteoconductive composite scaffold that promotes uniform cell seeding, cell development, and tissue creation. When coupled with collagen, PLLA, CS, and gelatin, HA and Tri calcium Phosphate (TCP), the inorganic component of bone, are employed as scaffolding [53].

A 3D gel-printing method can be used to create an interconnected porous pure HA scaffold. According to Shao et al., the inclusion of HA-based nanocomposites constructions in bone TE can be accomplished by combining 3D printing and microwave sintering to create a hierarchical porous HA scaffold with micropores and macropores. Song et al. revealed that these hierarchical HA scaffolds can be easily incorporated with native bone [54]. Bone regeneration is being attempted in all parts of the body, and the important ones are discussed below:

5.1.1 Maxilla

Trauma, defects, and cosmetic issues in the maxillofacial region necessitate bone tissue engineering. For bone regeneration, having an adequate scaffold is critical. Osteoinductive growth factors, such as BMP-2 and BMP-7, which are present in extracts of demineralized freeze-dried bone, can also be used to induce osteogenic cartilage periodontal attachment bone cementum hydroxyapatite in tissue engineering. After a trauma or tumor removal, HA and associated materials are utilized to repair a damaged maxilla. To fill the deficiencies, granular versions of HA and TCP are utilized, which shows improvement in bone regeneration in that area. Polymer scaffolds loaded with HA and TCP are also employed to promote tissue regeneration in the craniofacial region [55].

5.1.2 Mandible

Hydroxyapatite (HA) can also be utilized to regenerate mandibular bone. A lesion in the rabbit mandibular bone was created in an *in vivo* investigation and filled with porous Poly Methyl Methacrylate (PMMA) with or without HA. A new bone formed 12 weeks after implantation with no other surrounding tissue infection. The findings indicated that injectable porous PMMA-HA could be a reasonable solution for craniofacial bone regeneration. Nanocrystalline HA (HA-SiO) was employed to regenerate a mandibular bone defect in another animal investigation. The study found that HA accelerated the production of new bone tissue and had a high osteogenic potential. In clinical research, HA has also been utilized to treat a mandibular bone deformity. The magnesium-enriched HA was employed as a substitute in a mandibular bone defect caused by ameloblastoma excision in the study, and it was found to be effective in bone regeneration [56].

5.1.3 Alveolar bone

Periodontitis can cause damage to the alveolar bone that supports the teeth. The defective bone could be treated with tissue engineering or regenerative medicine. By providing a proper structural foundation, materials for a bone graft can induce bone healing. Rats had their alveolar bone defects repaired using a composite material made of HA. The new alveolar bone regenerated with good mechanical strength, biocompatibility, and a faster bone remodeling process, according to the researchers [57].

5.1.4 Calvarium

For the restoration of calvarial bone deformities, various materials have been proposed. In the seventeenth century, a gold plate was used to repair a calvarial defect for the first time. Other materials used in the previous century included tantalum, silver, titanium, and stainless steel. HA has been proposed as the most suitable biomaterial for the construction of biocomposite scaffolds for bone regeneration because of its superior osteoconductive and osteoinductive capabilities [58].

5.2 Periodontal tissue regeneration

Restoring periodontal tissues to their former shape and function is a difficult task. In a canine model with a labial alveolar bone defect, Liu et al. investigated the periodontal regeneration potential of collagen-HA scaffolds combined with bone marrow mesenchymal stem cells. The authors demonstrated that collagen-HA scaffolds supported periodontal tissue regeneration with no abnormal events occurring throughout the regeneration process, implying that collagen-HA scaffolds provide a biocompatible environment for periodontal regeneration. In another work, the nanoparticle HA was employed to promote the proliferation and differentiation of primary periodontal ligament cells (PDLC). When compared to the control group, HA brings extensive PDLC proliferation and alkaline phosphatase activity, suggesting that HA could be employed as a bioresorbable agent in osseous reconstruction [59].

5.3 Temporomandibular joint

The TMJ is a joint that connects the temporal bone to the mandibular condyle and is commonly damaged. TMJ traumatic abnormalities are divided into three categories:

"fracture, mandibular dislocation, and subluxation," which cause pain during necessary oral functions. Because there are few therapies for severe TMJ illnesses, there has been a surge in interest in regenerative techniques. TMJ regeneration has been studied by Mehrotra et al. Their research found that HA-enhanced collagen scaffolds facilitated the regeneration of entire TMJ condyles in adolescents and children with TMJ ankyloses. For the replacement of the mandibular condyle, a customized 3D polyamide implant-coated nano-HA can be planned and produced. The use of such materials in a patient has been shown to have favorable clinical consequences [60].

5.4 Cartilage

Proteoglycans, glycosaminoglycans, collagen fibers, and elastin make up the matrix of cartilage. Articular cartilage injuries are prevalent, and traumatic cartilage has limited healing and regeneration capability. Unfortunately, due to its limited ability to heal, articular cartilage lesions or injuries are difficult to heal, and artificial cartilage is necessary in the clinic. Articular cartilage grafting has been established in the literature to be a promising therapy option for these injuries [61]. The researchers discovered that HA stimulates chondrocytes to secrete the calcified cartilage matrix both *in vitro* and *in vivo* [62]. For cartilage repair, 3D printing may be utilized to build constructs with high structural complexity and flexibility, such as hydrogels, which offer the benefit of personalized precise customization, allowing the construct to match perfectly with the faulty surface. It has been established that HA-based nanocomposite structures can be used in cartilage TE.

5.5 Dentin

Dentin regeneration demands a proper scaffold system and an inductive microenvironment. In orthopedics and dentistry, HA was the most commonly used substance. HA is utilized not just in dental fillings and cement, but also in a variety of toothpaste that works as a polisher to reduce biofilm build-up on teeth. Dentin remineralization can be stimulated by advancements in dental materials that lead to the production of nHA particles [63]. nHA is a great source of free calcium and is an important factor in the prevention of dental caries and erosion. As a result, nHA is regarded to be a promising hard tissue engineering candidate [61]. The effect of HA particles of various sizes on the proliferation of pre-odontoblast cells (MDPC-23) has also been studied. The researchers also discovered that the size of HA particles is inversely related to cell proliferation. According to these findings, nHA could be a beneficial substitution for odontoblast cell proliferation [63].

5.6 Cementum

Cementum is a mineralized, avascular tissue that covers the surface of the root and creates the interface between the dentin and the periodontal ligament. Varying cementum has different proportionate compositions of chemical components. Cementum has a biological component that is identical to the bone, according to previous research. In the cementum, HA is a key inorganic component that is abundant (approximately 50%). The predominant components of the remaining organic matrix are proteoglycans, glycoproteins, and collagens [62, 64]. Periodontal infections or accidental damage can cause periodontal tissue degeneration, which can lead to teeth loosening and affect oral function. Cementum regeneration has been accomplished with HA based on a few studies. Mao et al. investigated the effect of HA bioceramics with a micro-nano-hybrid surface (mnHA) on human periodontal ligament stem cell adhesion, growth, and cementoblast differentiation. The findings showed that mnHA bioceramics stimulated cell proliferation, cell adhesion, alkaline phosphatase activity, and the expression of cementoblast differentiation markers such as cementum attachment protein and cementum protein [64].

5.7 3D printing of HA nanocomposites for dental applications

3D printing for dental applications has developed significantly in recent years, particularly in the fields of oral and maxillofacial surgery, endodontics, orthodontics, prosthodontics, and periodontics. The potential for personalized dental solutions promotes the use of 3D printing in this field. Dental prostheses and crowns are frequently made of metal, ceramic, and polymer-based materials. 3D printing is indeed being used to restore lost teeth. To assure a denser and more compact construction, the mechanical qualities of prosthodontic constructs must be addressed, and porosity difficulties must be avoided. Ink-jet printing, rather than SLS or SLA printing, can produce a denser and more compact structure. Controlling infection is said to be critical to the efficacy of apical surgery of root canal-treated teeth. However, because HA lacks bactericidal characteristics, antibacterial HA-based nanocomposites can prevent the growth of microorganisms in the root canal [65].

5.8 Drug delivery applications

For more precise and long-lasting drug release, HA has been combined with biopolymer (e.g., alginate) matrices. Venkata Subbu et al. [66], for example, placed the antibiotic ciprofloxacin onto a nano-HA composite using alginate. The medication was pre-adsorbed onto the ceramic particle before the composite was formed in their investigation. They discovered that integrating HA-based nanocomposites into ciprofloxacin-loaded HA increased the duration of ciprofloxacin release when compared to ciprofloxacin-loaded HA alone. In conclusion, the importance of HA-composites cannot be underestimated. Furthermore, recent studies from 2021 have shown that they can be used in human investigations. Kim and Kim, for example, used 3D strontium-substituted HA (Sr-HA) ceramic scaffolds in human cells to stimulate fast cell proliferation, osteogenic differentiation, and cellular mineralization. They used Sr-HA scaffolds as new bone graft alternatives in people and confirmed their effectiveness. Based on the reported success, it is expected that future research will focus on the use of HA-composites in people. The next section discusses what the future holds for HA composite applications in TE [66].

5.9 Future horizons

The use of nanotechnology in the manufacturing of HA is very beneficial. Since natural raw materials are used, HA production will be cost-effective in the near future. Cell culture, drug delivery, antibody purification, catheters, and engineered artificial organs constructed of HA composites are all interesting advancements for HA. Given the utility of HA-based nanocomposites in drug delivery, the scientists speculate that future applications for HA-based nanocomposites in the delivery of gene modifiers and targeted nutrition may be possible. Clearly, in the future, such technologies will allow for advanced and targeted cell and tissue transformations. In addition, various features of HA-based composites, such as printability, appropriate mechanical strength, biodegradation, and biocompatibility, will make it easier to use 3D printing to build on-demand, highly individualized complicated designs at low costs in the future. Recognizing that vascularization is critical for tissue regeneration and that functional vascularization of the biological scaffold is challenging to achieve with current 3D printing technologies, extrusion-based printing can be employed to provide the required structural integrity of the final result. The development of HA-based nanocomposites employing 3D printing in the future will address the vascularization issues stated above. However, a better understanding of the complex biological system is still required, and customized scaffolds created with 3D printing technology must be further developed with an increase in processing speed while avoiding mistakes and errors, as the printing process is not automated. In summary, we will be able to build better composites in the future if we can completely grasp the process of HA response to various cells and the signals they trigger. Cells respond differently depending on their microenvironment. Furthermore, the advancement of materials and 3D printing techniques is expected to lead to the development of HA-based nanocomposites for future clinical applications [67].

6. Conclusion

Despite extensive and new research into the treatment, critical-sized bone lesions are becoming more common and remain a significant barrier for tissue engineers. Desirable mechanical qualities merged into single tissue-engineered constructions as scaffold fabrication has increasingly aimed to include composite materials with greater bioactivity. As a result, several effective bone and cartilage structures with therapeutic application have been produced, with ceramic and polymer composites having excellent success. In the future, it will be essential to achieve even closer replication of natural mechanical and biochemical stimuli that cells are exposed to, as well as increased construct vascularization, to maximize osteogenesis and chondrogenesis. 3D bio-fabrication and bioprinting technologies provide ever-increasing precision in constructing microarchitecture. When combined with the growing number of bioactive materials, growth factors, functionalization processes, and biomimetic scaffold designs available, the future potential for constructing sophisticated BTE scaffolds suited to patient-specific applications is enormous. This gives hope for the treatment of several challenging illnesses, such as osteonecrosis, osteoporosis, and severe bone abnormalities. As manufacturing methods advance, it is believed that in the future, treatment personalized to the individual patient can be produced in a more cost-effective and efficient manner.

Author details

Senny Thomas Parackal[1*], Jose Paul[2], Johnson Dlima[2], Puthiya Veettil Darshana[2], Alenya Mary Pyas[3], Chamalayil Abdulrahman Sayed Mohammed Jiffry[2] and Sruthi K. Nair[2]

1 Comprehensive Dental Clinic, Annoor Dental College, India

2 Department of Periodontics, Annoor Dental College, India

3 Department of Periodontics, Indira Gandhi College of Dental Sciences, Kothamangalam, India

*Address all correspondence to: drsenny31@gmail.com

References

[1] Neira IS, Guitián F, Taniguchi T, Watanabe T, Yoshimura M. Hydrothermal synthesis of hydroxyapatite whiskers with sharp faceted hexagonal morphology. Journal of Materials Science. 2008;**43**(7):2171-2178

[2] Deb P, Barua E, Das Lala S, Deoghare AB. Synthesis of hydroxyapatite from Labeo rohita fish scale for biomedical application. Materials Today: Proceedings. 2019;**15**:277-283

[3] Varadavenkatesan T, Vinayagam R, Pai S, Kathirvel B, Pugazhendhi A, Selvaraj R. Synthesis, biological and environmental applications of hydroxyapatite and its composites with organic and inorganic coatings. Progress in Organic Coating. 2021;**151**:106056

[4] Ito Y, Hasuda H, Kamitakahara M, Ohtsuki C, Tanihara M, Kang I-K, et al. A composite of hydroxyapatite with electrospun biodegradable nanofibers as a tissue engineering material. Journal of Bioscience and Bioengineering. 2005;**100**:43-49

[5] Nair M, Nancy D, Krishnan AG, Anjusree GS, Vadukumpully S, Nair SV. Graphene oxide nanoflakes incorporated gelatin-hydroxyapatite scaffolds enhance osteogenic differentiation of human mesenchymal stem cells. Nanotechnology. 2015;**26**:161001

[6] Nosrati H, Sarraf Mamoory R, Svend Le DQ, Bünger CE. Fabrication of gelatin/hydroxyapatite/3D-graphene scaffolds by a hydrogel 3D-printing method. Materials Chemistry and Physics. 2020;**239**:122305

[7] Strobel LA, Rath SN, Maier AK, Beier JP, Arkudas A, Greil P, et al. Induction of bone formation in biphasic calcium phosphate scaffolds by bone morphogenetic protein-2 and primary osteoblasts. Journal of Tissue Engineering and Regenerative Medicine. 2014;**8**:176-185

[8] Woesz A, Rumpler M, Stampfl J, Varga F, Fratzl-Zelman N, Roschger P, et al. Towards bone replacement materials from calcium phosphates via rapid prototyping and ceramic gelcasting. Materials Science and Engineering: C. 2005;**25**:181-186

[9] Le Guéhennec L, Van Hede D, Plougonven E, Nolens G, Verlée B, De Pauw MC, et al. In vitro and in vivo biocompatibility of calcium-phosphate scaffolds three-dimensional printed by stereolithography for bone regeneration. Journal of Biomedial Materials Research Part A. 2020;**108**:412-425

[10] Milazzo M, Contessi Negrini N, Scialla S, Marelli B, Farè S, Danti S, et al. Additive manufacturing approaches for hydroxyapatite-reinforced composites. Advanced Functional Materials. Aug 2019;**29**(35):1903055

[11] Sun L, Parker ST, Syoji D, Wang X, Lewis JA, Kaplan DL. Direct-write assembly of 3D silk/hydroxyapatite scaffolds for bone co-cultures. Advanced Healthcare Materials. 2012;**1**:729-735

[12] Keriquel V, Oliveira H, Remy M, Ziane S, Delmond S, Rousseau B, et al. In situ printing of mesenchymal stromal cells, by laser-assisted bioprinting, for in vivo bone regeneration applications. Scientific Reports. 2017;**7**(1):1778

[13] Balasubramanian V, Herranz-Blanco B, Almeida PV, Hirvonen J, Santos HA. Multifaceted polymersome platforms: Spanning

from self-assembly to drug delivery and protocells. Progress in Polymer Science. 2016;**60**:51-85

[14] Koons GL, Diba M, Mikos AG. Materials design for bone-tissue engineering. Nature Reviews Materials. Aug 2020;**5**(8):548-603

[15] Samadikuchaksaraei A, Gholipourmalekabadi M, Erfani Ezadyar E, Azami M, Mozafari M, Johari B, et al. Fabrication and In vivo evaluation of an osteoblast-conditioned nano-hydroxyapatite/gelatine composite scaffold for bone tissue regeneration. Journal of Biomedial Materials Research Part A. 2016;**104**:2001-2010

[16] Wang L, Fang M, Xia YJ, Hou JX, Nan XR, Zhao Z, et al. Preparation and biological properties of silk fibroin/nanohydroxyapatite/graphene oxide scaffolds with an oriented channel-like structure. RSC Advances. 2020;**10**:10118-10128

[17] Kundu B, Rajkhowa R, Kundu SC, Wang X. Silk fibroin biomaterials for tissue regenerations. Advanced Drug Delivery Reviews. 2013;**65**:457-470

[18] He S, Timmer MD, Yaszemski MJ, Yasko AW, Engel PS, Mikos AG. Synthesis of biodegradable poly(propylene fumarate) networks with poly(propylene fumarate)-diacylate macromers as crosslinking agents and characterization of their degradation products. Polymer. 2001;**42**:1251-1260

[19] Lee JW, Ahn G, Kim DS, Cho DW. Development of nano- and microscale composite 3D scaffolds using PPF/DEF-HA and micro-stereolithography. Microelectronic Engineering. 2009;**86**:1465-1467

[20] Chirila TV, Suzuki S, Bray LJ, Barnett NL, Harkin DG. Evaluation of silk sericin as a biomaterial: In vitro growth of human corneal limbal epithelial cells on Bombyx mori sericin membranes. Progress in Biomaterials. 2013;**2**:1-10

[21] Mondal M, Trivedy K, Nirmal KS. The silk proteins, sericin and fibroin in silkworm, Bombyx mori Linn.—A review. Caspian Journal of Environmental Sciences. 2007;**5**:63-76

[22] Liu H, Li X, Zhou G, Fan H, Fan Y. Electrospun sulfated silk fibroin nanofibrous scaffolds for vascular tissue engineering. Biomaterials. 2011;**32**:3784-3793

[23] Favi PM, Ospina SP, Kachole M, Gao M, Atehortua L, Webster TJ. Preparation and characterization of biodegradable nano hydroxyapatite–bacterial cellulose composites with well-defined honeycomb pore arrays for bone tissue engineering applications. Cellulose. Apr 2016;**23**:1263-1282

[24] Venkatesan J, Bhatnagar I, Manivasagan P, Kang KH, Kim SK. Alginate composites for bone tissue engineering: A review. International Journal of Biological Macromolecules. 2015;**72**:269-281

[25] Domenech M, Polocorrales L, Ramirezvick JE, Freytes DO. TE strategies for myocardial regeneration: Acellular versus cellular scaffolds? Tissue Engineering. Part B, Reviews. 2016;**22**:438-458

[26] Hu Y, Wang J, Li X, Hu X, Zhou W, Dong X, et al. Facile preparation of bioactive nanoparticle/poly(ε-caprolactone) hierarchical porous scaffolds via 3D printing of high internal phase Pickering emulsions. Journal of Colloid and Interface Science. 2019;**545**:104-115

[27] Peter SJ, Miller ST, Zhu G, Yasko AW, Mikos AG. In vivo degradation of a poly(propylene fumarate)/β-tricalcium phosphate injectable composite scaffold. Journal of Biomedical Materials Research. 1998;**41**:1-7

[28] Lal B, Ghosh M, Agarwal B, Gupta D, Roychoudhury A. A novel economically viable solution for 3D printing-assisted cranioplast fabrication. British Journal of Neurosurgery. 2020;**34**:280-283

[29] Du GL, Nie L, Gao GR, Sun YN, Hou RX, Zhang H, et al. Tough and biocompatible hydrogels based on In situ interpenetrating networks of dithiol-connected graphene oxide and poly(vinyl alcohol). ACS Applied Materials & Interfaces. 2015;7:3003-3008

[30] Nie L, Li XC, Wang Z, Hu KH, Cai RH, Li P, et al. In vitro biomineralization on poly(vinyl alcohol)/biphasic calcium phosphate hydrogels. Bioinspired, Biomimetic and Nanobiomaterials. 2020;**9**:122-128

[31] Le Fer G, Luo YY, Becker ML. Poly(propylene fumarate) stars, using architecture to reduce the viscosity of 3D printable resins. Polymer Chemistry. 2019;**10**:4655-4664

[32] Lee KW, Wang S, Dadsetan M, Yaszemski MJ, Lu L. Enhanced cell ingrowth and proliferation through three-dimensional nanocomposite scaffolds with controlled pore structures. Biomacromolecules. 2010;**11**:682

[33] Asran AS, Henning S, Michler GH. Polyvinyl alcohol–collagen–hydroxyapatite biocomposite nanofibrous scaffold: Mimicking the key features of natural bone at the nanoscale level. Polymer. 2010;**51**:868-876

[34] Ferraz MP, Monteiro FJ, Manuel CM. Hydroxyapatite nanoparticles: A review of preparation methodologies. Journal of Applied Biomaterials & Biomechanics. 2004;**2**:74-80

[35] Zebarjad SM, Sajjadi SA, Sdrabadi TE, Yaghmaei A, Naderi B. A study on mechanical properties of PMMA/hydroxyapatite nanocomposite. Engineering. 2011;**3**:795-801

[36] Cai X, Tong H, Shen X, Chen W, Yan J, Hu J. Preparation and characterization of homogeneous chitosan-polylactic acid/hydroxyapatite nanocomposite for bone tissue engineering and evaluation of its mechanical properties. Acta Biomaterialia. 2009;**5**:2693-2703

[37] Wolfe PS, Sell SA, Bowlin GL. Natural and synthetic scaffolds. In: Tissue Engineering: From Lab to Clinic. Berlin, Heidelberg: Springer; 24 Nov 2010. pp. 41-67

[38] Hoyer B, Bernhardt A, Heinemann S, Stachel I, Meyer M, Gelinsky M. Biomimetically mineralized salmon collagen scaffolds for application in bone tissue engineering. Biomacromolecules. 2012;**13**(4):1059-1066

[39] White RA, Weber JN, White EW. Replamine form: A new process for preparing porous ceramics, metal and polymer prosthetic materials. Science. 1972;**176**:922-924

[40] Danilchenko SN, Kalinkevich OV, Pogorelov MV, Kalinkevich AN, Sklyar AM, Kalinichenko TG, et al. Characterization and in vivo evaluation of chitosan-hydroxyapatite bone scaffolds made by one step coprecipitation method. Journal of Biomedical Materials Research. Part A. 2011;**96**:639-647

[41] Ma XY, Feng YF, Ma ZS, Li X, Wang J, Wang L, et al. The promotion

of osteointegration under diabetic conditions using chitosan/hydroxyapatite composite coating on porous titanium surfaces. Biomaterials. 2014;**35**:7259-7270

[42] Stanford ECC. Improvements in the manufacture of useful products from seaweeds. British Patent. 1881;**142** [Google Scholar]

[43] Toole BP. Hyaluronan: From extracellular glue to pericellular cue. Nature Reviews. Cancer. 2004;**4**(7):528-539

[44] Misch CE, Qu Z, Bidez MW. Mechanical properties of trabecular bone in the human mandible: Implications for dental implant treatment planning and surgical placement. Journal of Oral and Maxillofacial Surgery. 1999;**57**(6):700-706

[45] Bhumiratana S, Grayson WL, Castaneda A, Rockwood DN, Gil ES, Kaplan DL, et al. Nucleation and growth of mineralized bone matrix on silk-hydroxyapatite composite scaffolds. Biomaterials. 2011;**32**:2812-2812

[46] Ivanov AN, Kozadaev MN, Bogomolova NV, Matveeva OV, Puchin'yan MD, Norkin IA, et al. Biocompatibility of polycaprolactone and hydroxyapatite matrices in vivo. Cell and Tissue Biology. 2015;**9**(5):422-429

[47] Shishatskaya EI, Khlusov IA, Volova TG. A hybrid PHB hydroxyapatite composite for biomedical application: Production, in vitro and in vivo investigation. Journal of Biomaterials Science. Polymer Edition. 2006;**17**(5):481-498

[48] Nie L, Chen D, Suo J, Zou P, Feng S, Yang Q, et al. Physicochemical characterization and biocompatibility in vitro of biphasic calcium phosphate/polyvinyl alcohol scaffolds prepared by freeze-drying method for bone tissue engineering applications. Colloids and Surfaces. B, Biointerfaces. 2012;**100**:169e

[49] Paul W, Sharma CP. Development of porous spherical hydroxyapatite granules: Application towards protein delivery. Journal of Materials Science. Materials in Medicine. 1999;**10**(7):383-388

[50] Liao SS, Cui FZ, Zhang W, Feng QL. Hierarchically biomimetic bone scaffold materials: Nano-HA/collagen/PLA composite. Journal of Biomedical Materials Research. Part B, Applied Biomaterials. 2004;**69**(2):158-165

[51] Fisher PD, Venugopal G, Milbrandt TA, Hilt JZ, Puleo DA. Hydroxyapatite-reinforced in situ forming PLGA systems for intraosseous injection. Journal of Biomedical Materials Research. Part A. 2015;**103**(7):2365-2373

[52] Huang YX, Ren J, Chen C, Ren TB, Zhou XY. Preparation and properties of poly(lactide-co-glycolide) (PLGA)/nano-hydroxyapatite (NHA) scaffolds by thermally induced phase separation and rabbit MSCs culture on scaffolds. Journal of Biomaterials Applications. 2008;**22**(5):409-432

[53] Zhang R, Ma PX. Porous poly (l-lactic acid)/apatite composites created by biomimetic process. Journal of Biomedical Materials Research. 1999;**45**:285-293

[54] Pei X, Ma L, Zhang BQ, Sun JX, Sun Y, Fan YJ, et al. Creating hierarchical porosity hydroxyapatite scaffolds with osteoinduction by three-dimensional printing and microwave sintering. Biofabrication. 14 Nov 2017;**9**(4):045008

[55] Petite H, Vandamme K, Monfoulet L, Logeart-Avramoglou D. Strategies for improving the efficacy of bioengineered bone constructs: A

perspective. Osteoporosis International. 2011;**22**:2017-2021

[56] Broggini N, Bosshardt DD, Jensen SS, Bornstein MM, Wang CC, Buser D. Bone healing around nanocrystalline hydroxyapatite, deproteinized bovine bone mineral, biphasic calcium phosphate, and autogenous bone in mandibular bone defects. Journal of Biomedical Materials Research. Part B, Applied Biomaterials. 2015;**103**:1478-1487

[57] Subramaniam S, Fang Y-H, Sivasubramanian S, Lin F-H, Lin C-P. Hydroxyapatite-calcium sulfate-hyaluronic acid composite encapsulated with collagenase as bone substitute for alveolar bone regeneration. Biomaterials. 2016;**74**:99-108

[58] Jang J-H, Castano O, Kim H-W. Electrospun materials as potential platforms for bone tissue engineering. Advanced Drug Delivery Reviews. 2009;**61**:1065-1083

[59] Liu Z, Yin X, Ye Q, He W, Ge M, Zhou X, et al. Periodontal regeneration with stem cells-seeded collagen-hydroxyapatite scaffold. Journal of Biomaterials Applications. 2016;**31**:121-131

[60] Li J, Hsu Y, Luo E, Khadka A, Hu J. Computer-aided design and manufacturing and rapid prototyped nanoscale hydroxyapatite/polyamide (n-HA/PA) construction for condylar defect caused by mandibular angle ostectomy. Aesthetic Plastic Surgery. 2011;**35**:636-664

[61] Curl WW, Krome J, Gordon ES, Rushing J, Smith BP, Poehling GG. Cartilage injuries: A review of 31,516 knee arthroscopies. Arthroscopy: The Journal of Arthroscopic & Related Surgery. 1 Aug 1997;**13**(4):456-460

[62] You F, Chen X, Cooper D, Chang T, Eames BF. Homogeneous hydroxyapatite/alginate composite hydrogel promotes calcified cartilage matrix deposition with potential for three-dimensional bioprinting. Biofabrication. 2018;**11**:015015

[63] Teotia AK, Raina DB, Singh C, Sinha N, Isaksson H, TaGil M, et al. Nano-hydroxyapatite bone substitute functionalized with bone active molecules for enhanced cranial bone regeneration. ACS Applied Materials & Interfaces. 2017;**9**:6816-6828

[64] Bosshardt DD, Selvig KA. Dental cementum: The dynamic tissue covering of the root. Periodontology 2000. 1997;**13**:41-75

[65] Shah P, Chong BS. 3D imaging, 3D printing and 3D virtual planning in endodontics. Clinical Oral Investigations. 2018;**22**:641-654

[66] Venkatasubbu GD, Ramasamy S, Ramakrishnan V, Kumar J. Hydroxyapatite-alginate nanocomposite as drug delivery matrix for sustained release of ciprofloxacin. Journal of Biomedical Nanotechnology. 2011;7:759-767

[67] Tappa K, Jammalamadaka U. Novel biomaterials used in medical 3D printing techniques. Journal of Functional Biomaterials. 2018;**9**:17

Chapter 4

Toxicity of Natural Hydroxyapatite

Saumya John, Rakhi Manoharan, Kavya Suresh, Lekshmi Mini, Nibu Varghese, Sajith Vellapally and Nebu George Thomas

Abstract

Hydroxyapatite (HA) has been extensively researched in bone regeneration procedures for its close similarity with natural bone in composition and also due to its osteoconductive and bone healing properties. Natural hydroxyapatite (NHA) is dissimilar to its synthetic counterpart. It has a slight difference in the calcium phosphate ratio and contains carbonate groups and some trace elements, which makes it a more viable material as a substitute for bone. Biowaste is a huge environmental concern. NHA is generated from biowaste of mostly poultry and marine origin. Hence, its proven biocompatibility would advocate the translation of this knowledge to clinical practice for bone regenerative procedures. *In vitro* biocompatibility of NHA from various sources has been reported. Also, *in vivo* studies, including implantation studies, have been carried out to certify the biological safety of NHA. Various authors have stated that the preparation technique (which influences features of NHA), degradation characteristics, and resulting tissue response of NHA are also satisfactory. This chapter elaborates on the toxicity assessment *in vitro*, and *in vivo* and hence the biocompatibility of NHA obtained from various sources.

Keywords: hydroxyapatite, natural hydroxyapatite, egg shell-based hydroxyapatite, fish scale derived hydroxyapatite, MTT assay, marine hydroxyapatite

1. Introduction

Hydroxyapatite (HA) resembles bone minerals in terms of bioactivity, mechanical characteristics, and composition; hence, it is frequently employed as a bone substitute [1, 2]. Recently, hydroxyapatite nanoparticles have been used for the purpose of drug delivery, where they serve as vehicles for pharmaceutical molecules, bioimaging molecules, and other therapeutic agents. It is asserted that these particle drug delivery methods have improved bioavailability, predictable treatment outcomes, higher efficacy and safety, and the potential for controlled release.

Although NHA is demonstrating considerable promise in the biomedical field, careful consideration of its possible toxicity is necessary before it can be considered a viable option for medical application in the broader human population [3, 4].

2. Safety evaluation of NHA

The safety evaluation of NHA includes reports on its *in vitro* response in cell-culture followed by *in vivo* response to short term and long term presence of NHA in the various animal models [1, 3–5]. The sequence of toxicity evaluation tests for NHA reported in literature has been represented in **Figure 1**.

2.1 *In vitro* toxicity evaluation of NHA

2.1.1 Cytotoxicity

It is crucial to assess in vitro cytotoxicity of medical devices to understand their impact on cell functions. Various authors have studied cytotoxicity of NHA in vitro prior to its applications in bone regeneration [3–5]. MTT assay (based on cell culture) is considered as the most preferred methods to carry out in cytotoxicity assessment [5]. Only the viable cells will have mitochondrial succinate dehydrogenase to convert the MTT to formazan crystals. Various cell lines, preferably osteoblast based are utilized to carry out MTT assay to clearly identify response of NHA on osteoblast cell lineage. DNA quantification assay is also carried out to analyze the DNA changes in these cells if they correspond with healthy cells.

Oyster (Crassostrea angulate) shells based on their microporous scaffold-like form have been used to create NHA scaffolds. Osteoblast lineage cells when seeded in these scaffolds followed by their proliferation was compared to synthetic HA scaffolds using MTT assay. NHA scaffolds yielded better results than synthetic HA scaffolds [4].

NHA was extracted using fishbone of Tuna (Thunnus thynnus) and from sword fish (Xiphias gladius) [3]. The frozen bones were cleaned, dried, calcined (at 600 and 950°C) and milled. Both the NHA extracts were incorporated in mouse calvarial cell culture. Following MTT assay was found to be nontoxic for 100% extract concentration.

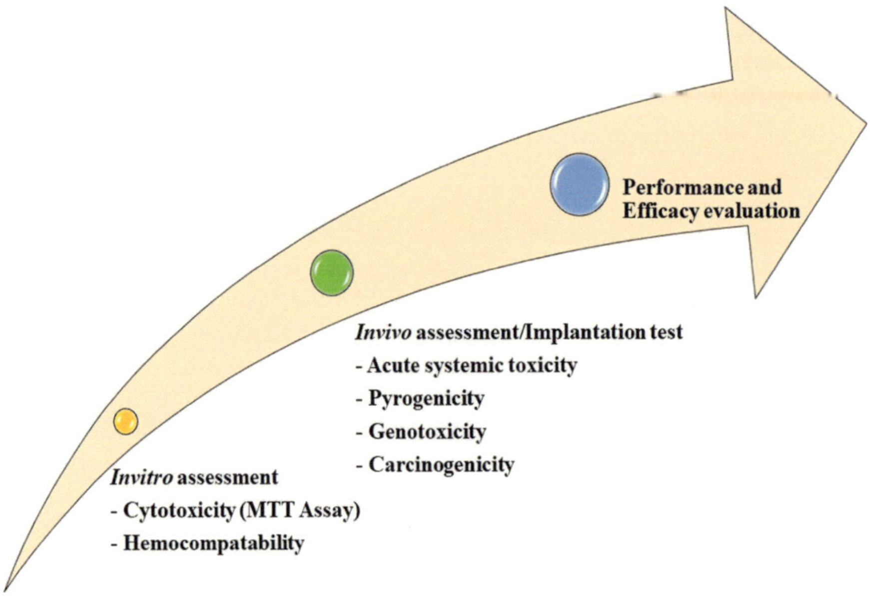

Figure 1.
The sequence of toxicity evaluation tests carried out for NHA reported in literature.

Osteoblast (MG63) and fibroblast (NIH3T3) cells were cultured in Mercenaria mercenaria seashells extract. Following MTT assay was found to be noncytotoxic [6].

Shamsuria [7] assessed the *in vitro* cytotoxicity of natural corals in human osteoblast cells following extraction in complete culture medium. After a 72-h incubation time, the viability of the osteoblast CRL-1543 was evaluated and compared to a negative control using the neutral red assay using a spectrophotometer set at 540 nm. The outcomes demonstrated that the materials were not cytotoxic. Following 72 h of incubation, hydroxyapatite revealed 123% viable cells, Natural Coral revealed 99.43%, and Polyhydroxybutarate revealed 176.75%. The cytotoxicity test in this investigation primarily focused on the chemicals that leached out of the biomaterial. The outcomes demonstrated the materials' lack of toxicity and their ability to support biofunctional cell growth.

Prado et al. [8] evaluated NHA powders using fish waste (Micropogonias furnieri). It was incubated (0.05 g/ml concentration) in osteoblast cell lines placed in αMEM culture medium with 10% fetal bovine serum and 1% antibiotic. *In vitro* cytotoxicity was analyzed based on its incorporation in the cells using Alamar Blue assay. Pre-osteoblast cells on 3rd and 5th day demonstrated reduced cytotoxicity. Also DNA quantification revealed reduced concentration and quantitative RT-PCR did not reveal any significant difference between the control and test group.

Panda et al. [9] prepared NHA powder obtained from fish scales (fresh water fish-Labeo rohita and Catla catla). MTT assay was carried out using Mesenchymal stem cells derived from cord blood. Cell viability was found to be enhanced on the 5th day. DNA quantification assay revealed increase in DNA content.

Lee et al. [10] fabricated chitosan based micro- and nano-hydroxyapaptite as scaffolds for bone tissue engineering. *In vitro* cell viability and cell proliferation assay on osteoblast cell lines revealed the NHA to be biocompatible and promote cell growth.

Venkatesan et al. [11] isolated NHA from salmon fish bone. Cytotoxicity was assessed in cultured MSCs using MTT assay. Up to 100 μg/ml NHA was found to noncytotoxic to MSCs. Cell interactions observed using optical microscopy revealed no changes in MSCS incorporated with NHA.

Pon-on et al. [12] synthesized calcium phosphate of HA powder from the fish scales of *Probarbus jullieni*. Fish scale derived NHA was found to be biocompatible with osteoblast cell lines. The cells exhibited greater adhesion and spreadability on these fish scale-based NHA as compared to synthetic HA.

Shi et al. 2018 used mouse preosteoblast MC3T3-E1 in an alkaline phosphatase activity investigation and the MTT cell viability assay to assess the cytocompatibility of calcined nHAP [13]. According to the results of a cell experiment, nHAP derived from rainbow trout and salmon bones had superior biological compatibility than nHAP derived from cod bone and chemically synthesized HAP (cHAP). The inclusion of $CO3^{2-}$ and Mg^{2+} in the nHAP generated from rainbow trout and salmon bones is most likely to blame for this difference in element composition. As a result, the natural waste fish bone product (nHAP) derived from rainbow trout and salmon bones has a promising possibility for utilization as an alternative for biomaterial in bone tissue engineering and may be employed as hydroxyapatite.

2.1.2 Hemocompatibility test

Lu [14] carried out hemocompatibility test for nHA-chitosan composite in rabbit blood diluted with saline solution and assessed using spectrophotometer. It revealed good hemocompatibility.

2.2 In vivo toxicity evaluation of NHA

2.2.1 Implantation test

The most crucial factor in determining biocompatibility of a biomaterial is its response locally and systemically once implanted in *in vivo* models [1, 5]. It needs to be assessed for integration, or biodegradation within the animal models (ISO 10993-6, 2016) [1].

In vivo study on rat calvarial defects revealed chronic inflammatory infiltrate in response to nHA (from marine biowaste generated from *Micropogonias furnieri*), after the 7th and 15th day which was absent after 30 days of the implantation [8].

Strombus gigas (conch) shells and *Tridacna gigas* (Giant clam) shells were converted to NHA bone implants using hydrothermal method [15]. This was placed in femoral defects in rats to assess whether they can be used as block grafts for load-bearing areas. The study revealed good biocompatibility with definitive osseointegration for bulk shell derived NHA.

NHA derived from dolphin (*Neophocaena asiaeorientalis*) back bone was combined with poly-L-lactic acid (PLA) and compared with standard PLA [16]. Both were subcutaneously implanted to assess toxicity *in vivo*. There was no severe immunological response to this NHA composite in the subcutaneous tissues of the Sprague-Dawley rats.

Nandi et al synthesized NHA scaffolds from sea corals [17]. The *in vivo* tests were done in tibial defects in New Zealand white rabbits. Eighteen rabbits were divided into three groups. In the first group only coralline NHA implant was placed. In the second group insulin growth factor-1 was incorporated into the coralline NHA implant prior to placement. In the third group bone morphogenetic protein-2 was incorporated into the coralline NHA implants. After 90 days of implantation bone histology slides revealed healthy bone formation in all the groups however the quality of bone was the best in group two.

2.2.2 Acute systemic toxicity

Lu et al. [14] utilized hydroxyapatite from pig bones and combined with chitosan to form a composite bone graft material. The acute systemic toxicity was assessed in 30 Kumming rats after injecting the extract of the composite material. The mice in the experimental group did not show any signs of toxicity.

Lee [16] assessed a composite of NHA derived from dolphin backbone with PLA in Sprague-Dawley rats. After eight months systemic toxicity was assessed based on response in the liver and kidneys to the NHA based implant. There was no significant difference in the hepato- and nephro-toxicity indicators between the test and control groups after eight months.

2.2.3 Genotoxicity

Genotoxicity involves assessment of any mutations or chromosomal abnormalities in response to the medical device being tested [1, 5]. Genotoxicity testing is usually not carried out if the chemical characterization of extracts from the device has been already carried out. Also, if there is sufficient literature stating that the components of the device have been tested for genotoxicity these tests are not repeated for the device [1].

Yamamura et al. [18] synthesized hydroxyapatite from Whitemouth croaker (*Micropogonias furnieri*) fish waste. They carried out genotoxicity assessment after 30 days in the vital organs in Wistar rats following subcutaneous implantation of nHA in of the animals. NHA obtained was found to have no cytotoxicity and genotoxicity.

There are no reports till date on intracutaneous reactivity and skin sensitization assay.

2.2.4 Pyrogenicity test

Lu [14] examined the pyrogenicity of nHA-Chitosan composite in New Zealand rabbits. Rectal temperature was recorded ten minutes after injecting the extract in the ear vein. No significant variation in the body temperature of the rabbit was found.

2.2.5 Carcinogenicity assessment

Lu [14] assessed teratogenicity/mutagenicity of nHA-Chitosan using rabbit calvarial defect models. The graft material was placed in the defects and these were reassessed after six months and no genetic changes were found.

2.3 Performance and efficacy evaluation

Implantation test is crucial to determine the performance and efficacy of the medical device [1]. Biocompatibility and efficacy of the bone grafts can be evaluated simultaneously through critical size defects in animal models ISO10993-6 (2016) (FDA, 2016) [1]. As per the ISO guidelines these tests need to be carried out in identical test and control groups with minimum 10 implantation sites.

Similarly Prado et al. [8] evaluated the biological performance and biocompatibility of NHA simultaneously in rat calvarial defects. Runx-2 expression following immunohistochemistry was detected after 7th, 15th and 30th day indicative that the nHA might be osteoinductive in nature.

Oryan et al [19] evaluated salmon fish bone and demineralized bone matrix implanted in the radial bone defect model (murine study). Radiographic, histopathological and biochemical evaluation was found to be favorable. There was evidence of new bone formation on routine histopathological examination on 35th and 56th day postoperatively.

3. Toxicology aspects in major applications of natural hydroxyapatite

3.1 In membrane protein interactions

Xu et al. [20] studied the interaction of nanoscale hydroxyapatite with cytochrome c, a heme protein in the inner mitochondrial membrane, and hemoglobin, an iron-containing metalloprotein, in zebrafish embryonic development. Experimental results showed that the interaction was formed by intramolecular charge and hydrogen bond interactions. The two functional proteins are cross-linked by charge and hydrogen bond interactions between hydroxyapatite particles aggregated colloidally. Therefore, this study found hydroxyapatite can accumulate in larger particles around membrane proteins and is toxic to zebrafish embryo development.

3.2 In dentine surface coating

Nano-sized hydroxyapatite can be used as a coating material for the remineralization of caries dentin specimens [21]. This study found that dentin specimens could be effectively coated with hydroxyapatite and there was no evidence of toxicity. In addition to its nontoxic effects, hydroxyapatite also actively contributed to the viability of L929 fibroblasts and showed antibacterial effects against certain bacteria responsible for caries.

3.3 In bone marrow stem cells

Remya et al. [22], has studied the molecular toxicity of the hydroxyapatite nanoparticles using mouse bone marrow mesenchymal stem cells. The MTT assay showed that hydroxyapatite did not cause any kind of cytotoxicity up to 800 μg/ml. Moreover, when the oxidative stress induced apoptosis and the levels of reactive oxygen species generation were studied, it was giving a result which was not significantly different from the control group, which concludes the nontoxic or safe nature of hydroxy apatite especially in mesenchymal stem cells.

3.4 In bone tissue engineering scaffolds

Paras et al., 2020 performed a toxicological assessment of highly porous nano-hydroxyapatite-based scaffolds [23]. In vitro genotoxicity was measured using the Comet assay and evaluated for systemic subchronic toxicity by oral administration of nano calcium hydroxyapatite covered with a small scaffold layer for 120 days. These nanohydroxyapatite-based scaffolds had minimal risk, as evidenced by genotoxicity and systemic toxicity studies. No genotoxic effects were seen even at high concentrations of 50 mg nanohydroxyapatite scaffolds. In addition, daily oral administration of nanohydroxyapatite-based scaffolds at high concentrations over extended periods did not induce significant adverse changes in the internal organs of the test animals. This subacute, chronic toxicity study shows that this may be a promising advance in mimicking natural bone in terms of structural and mechanical properties.

3.5 Intravenously as a drug vehicle

In a study conducted by Liu et al. 2005 [24], hydroxyapatite solutions were injected intravenously into rabbits at different concentrations, and the response and viability of the rabbits were observed to study the effect of nanohydroxyapatite on living organs. Nanohydroxyapatite had no cumulative toxicity to rabbits and is considered to be safe. It can be intravenously administered with hydroxyapatite as a drug carrier at a low dose lower than the average lethal dose.

3.6 In bone grafting applications

Several studies demonstrated the ability of hydroxyapatite to generate a positive environment for facilitating new bone tissue growth and regeneration. It results in perfect incorporation of the graft without undergoing any development of severe immune response. Calcium hydroxyapatite-based bioceramics show excellent biocompatibility, corrosion resistance, and excellent compressive strength, making them good candidates for implants.

Natural hydroxyapatite is the most successful in bone graft applications due to its low toxicity and resemblance to the mineral bone, with properties that promote osseointegration and new bone formation processes. Rincón-López et al. 2018; showed that alternative allogeneic transplant materials derived from naturally occurring heterologous hydroxyapatite have been developed [25]. Heterologous bone graft materials can be used as fully crystalline, naturally porous, bovine-derived hydroxyapatite (all collagen protein removed) in a particle size range of 250–450 μm. Organic matter is previously been removed, but the bone microstructure is preserved. Hydroxyapatite has been used in a variety of biomedical applications because it is synthetically or naturally produced and has the ability to form a bone-like apatite layer primarily at the interface between bone tissues.

4. Conclusion

Various studies support the biocompatibility of natural hydroxyapatite and have concluded that it is appropriate for bone substitution. The biological waste fish bone products is suitable for the production of hydroxyapatite as part of bio-waste treatment, and the nHAP derived using rainbow trout and salmon remains has significant promise for usage as an implant product alternative in tissue engineering of bones. Bone tissue engineering has come up as a novel field in regenerative medicine and biomaterials have three-dimensional essential functions of cell adhesion, diffusion, proliferation, differentiation, and tissue formation. The application of hydroxyapatite nanoparticles in the biopolymer matrix enhances the mechanical strength and nano topographical characteristics which resembles the nanostructures of natural bone. Based on the reported studies, the integration of beneficial effects of natural absorbent polymers and nanoscale sized bioactive ceramic components has been found to be important for usage in bone regeneration. Natural hydroxyapatite is known for its biocompatibility, and bioactivity which is called as the ability to form direct chemical bonds with surrounding tissues, osteoconductive, nontoxicity, noninflammatory and nonimmunogenic properties. Therefore, natural hydroxyapatite is one of the ideal materials for bone tissue engineering due to its biocompatibility and mechanical strength.

Conflict of interest

The authors declare no conflict of interest.

Appendix and nomenclature

NHA natural hydroxyapatite

Author details

Saumya John[1*], Rakhi Manoharan[1], Kavya Suresh[1], Lekshmi Mini[1], Nibu Varghese[2], Sajith Vellapally[3] and Nebu George Thomas[1]

1 Department Periodontology, Pushpagiri College of Dental Sciences, Thiruvalla, India

2 MACFAST, Thiruvalla, India

3 Dental Biomaterials Research Chair, Dental health Department, College of Applied Medical Sciences, King Saud University, Riyadh, Saudi Arabia

*Address all correspondence to: drsaumyajohn85@gmail.com

References

[1] Health C for D and R. Use of International Standard ISO 10993-1, Biological Evaluation of Medical Devices. Part 1. Evaluation and Testing Within a Risk Management Process. Rockville, Maryland, USA: U.S. Food and Drug Administration—FDA; 2020 (cited 2022 Mar 20)

[2] Kavasi RM, Coelho CC, Platania V, Quadros PA, Chatzinikolaidou M. In vitro biocompatibility assessment of nano-hydroxyapatite. Nanomaterials (Basel). 2021;**11**(5):1152

[3] Boutinguiza M, Pou J, Comesaña R, Lusquiños F, de Carlos A, León B. Biological hydroxyapatite obtained from fish bones. Materials Science and Engineering C. 2012;**32**(3):478-486

[4] Borciani G, Fischetti T, Ciapetti G, Montesissa M, Baldini N, Graziani G. Marine biological waste as a source of hydroxyapatite for bone tissue engineering applications. Ceramics International. 2023;**49**(2):1572-1584

[5] Li W, Zhou J, Xu Y. Study of the in vitro cytotoxicity testing of medical devices. Biomedical Reports. 2015;**3**(5):617-620

[6] Pal A, Maity S, Chabri S, Bera S, Chowdhury AR, Das M, et al. Mechanochemical synthesis of nanocrystalline hydroxyapatite from Mercenaria clam shells and phosphoric acid. Biomedical Physics & Engineering Express. 2017;**3**(1):015010

[7] Shamsuria O, Fadilah AS, Asiah AB, Rodiah MR, Suzina AH, Samsudin AR. In vitro cytotoxicity evaluation of biomaterials on human osteoblast cells CRL-1543; hydroxyapatite, natural coral and polyhydroxybutarate. The Medical Journal of Malaysia. 2004;**59**(Suppl B):174-175

[8] JPdS P, Yamamura H, AMP M, PLM R, JLdS P, ACM R, et al. In vitro and in vivo biological performance of hydroxyapatite from fish waste. Journal of Materials Science: Materials in Medicine. 2021;**32**(9):109

[9] Panda NN, Pramanik K, Sukla LB. Extraction and characterization of biocompatible hydroxyapatite from fresh water fish scales for tissue engineering scaffold. Bioprocess and Biosystems Engineering. 2014;**37**(3):433-440

[10] Lee J, Baek S, Venkatesan J, Bhatnagar I, Chang H, Kim H, et al. In vivo study of chitosan-natural nano hydroxyapatite scaffolds for bone tissue regeneration. International Journal of Biological Macromolecules. 2014;**67**

[11] Venkatesan J, Lowe B, Manivasagan P, Kang KH, Chalisserry EP, Anil S, et al. Isolation and characterization of nano-hydroxyapatite from Salmon fish bone. Materials. 2015;**8**(8):5426-5439

[12] Pon-On W, Suntornsaratoon P, Charoenphandhu N, Thongbunchoo J, Krishnamra N, Tang IM. Hydroxyapatite from fish scale for potential use as bone scaffold or regenerative material. Materials Science and Engineering: C. 2016;**62**:183-189

[13] Shi P, Liu M, Fan F, Yu C, Lu W, Du M. Characterization of natural hydroxyapatite originated from fish bone and its biocompatibility with osteoblasts. Materials Science and Engineering: C, Materials for Biological Applications. 2018;**90**:706-712

[14] Lü X, Zheng B, Tang X, Zhao L, Lu J, Zhang Z, et al. In vitro biomechanical and biocompatible evaluation of natural hydroxyapatite/chitosan

composite for bone repair. Journal of Applied Biomaterials & Biomechanics. 2011;**9**(1):11-18

[15] Vecchio KS, Zhang X, Massie JB, Wang M, Kim CW. Conversion of bulk seashells to biocompatible hydroxyapatite for bone implants. Acta Biomaterialia. 2007;**3**(6):910-918

[16] Lee MR, Lee GW, Kim JE, Yun WB, Choi JY, Park JJ, et al. Biocompatibility of a PLA-based composite containing hydroxyapatite derived from waste bones of dolphin *Neophocaena asiaeorientalis*. Journal of the Australian Ceramic Society. 2019;**55**(1):269-279

[17] Nandi SK, Kundu B, Mukherjee J, Mahato A, Datta S, Balla VK. Converted marine coral hydroxyapatite implants with growth factors: In vivo bone regeneration. Materials Science and Engineering: C. 2015;**49**:816-823

[18] Yamamura H, da Silva VHP, Ruiz PLM, Ussui V, Lazar DRR, Renno ACM, et al. Physico-chemical characterization and biocompatibility of hydroxyapatite derived from fish waste. Journal of the Mechanical Behavior of Biomedical Materials. 2018;**80**:137-142

[19] Oryan A, Bigham-Sadegh A, Monazzah S. Fish bone versus fish demineralized bone matrix (vertebra) effects on healing of experimental radial defect in rat model. Comparative Clinical Pathology. 2016;**25**(5):981-985

[20] Xu Z, Zhang YL, Song C, Wu LL, Gao HW. Interactions of hydroxyapatite with proteins and its toxicological effect to zebrafish embryos development. PLoS One. 2012;**7**(4):e32818

[21] Erdem U, Dogan M, Metin AU, Baglar S, Turkoz MB, Turk M, et al. Hydroxyapatite-based nanoparticles as a coating material for the dentine surface: An antibacterial and toxicological effect. Ceramics International. 2020;**46**(1):270-280

[22] Remya NS, Syama S, Gayathri V, Varma HK, Mohanan PV. An in vitro study on the interaction of hydroxyapatite nanoparticles and bone marrow mesenchymal stem cells for assessing the toxicological behaviour. Colloids and Surfaces. B, Biointerfaces. 2014;**117**:389-397

[23] Paraš S, Trišić D, Mitrović Ajtić O, Prokić B, Drobne D, Živković S, et al. Toxicological profile of nanostructured bone substitute based on hydroxyapatite and poly(lactide-co-glycolide) after subchronic oral exposure of rats. Nanomaterials. 2020;**10**(5):918

[24] Liu LP, Xiao YB, Xiao ZW, Wang ZB, Li C, Gong X. Toxicity of hydroxyapatite nanoparticles on rabbits. Wei Sheng yan jiu= Journal of Hygiene Research. 2005;**34**(4):474-476

[25] Rincón-LópezJA, Hermann-MuñozJA, Giraldo-Betancur AL, De Vizcaya-Ruiz A, Alvarado-Orozco JM, Muñoz-Saldaña J. Synthesis, characterization and in vitro study of synthetic and bovine-derived hydroxyapatite ceramics: A comparison. Materials (Basel). 2018;**11**(3):333. DOI: 10.3390/ma11030333

Chapter 5

Novel Titanium Alloys for Tissue Engineering

Petrica Vizureanu, Madalina Simona Baltatu and Andrei Victor Sandu

Abstract

Taking into account the speed of industrial development and market request for novel biocompatible alloys, the urge of creating sustainable materials pushes the research forward. Among the many biomaterials that can be incorporated into the human body, in the class of metal alloys, titanium and titanium alloys are regarded as some of the most important biomaterials because of their resistance to the effects of body fluids, high tensile strength, flexibility, and corrosion resistance, as well as their unique combination of strength and biocompatibility. In present chapter several novel recipes for titanium alloys are presented and characterized (Ti-Mo-Si and Ti-Mo-Zr-Ta-Si systems).

Keywords: titanium alloys, high biocompatibility, low Young modulus, morphological characterization, biocompatibility assessment

1. Introduction

Biomaterials are substances that are utilized to replace a piece of a living system or work closely with a live tissue. Materials that come into touch with live tissues and their biological fluids might be natural, synthetic, or composite. Metals, polymers, ceramics, and composites are the four major categories into which biomaterials are categorized. They are utilized in the medical industry in a variety of forms, including complete pieces, particles/powders, fibers, thin films, thick coatings that are either porous or non-porous, etc. Implants and other medical devices range in size from a few nanometers to a few centimeters, with a variety of forms and geometries. Additionally, many biomaterials need their surfaces modified in order to provide the intended biological effects [1, 2].

Typically, biocompatible alloys are employed in bone replacement when we talk about them. Bone functions as an organ together with its numerous ancillary components, including connective tissue, cartilage, neuron, and vascular parts. They aid in protecting and supporting soft tissues while collaborating with skeletal muscles to enable movement of the body. Bones are rather hard structures, and they closely resemble one another in terms of shape and function [2]. Internal or external fixation is an element of the therapy for long bones since they are prone to damage. Another significant procedure where the bone has to absorb biomaterials is joint replacement.

The process of regeneration is interrupted by the bone's reaction to the biomaterial. However, because they are inert, materials placed in bone will cause local and systemic biological reactions. An adaptive and reactive process involving several factors will be triggered by host reactions to joint replacement and fixation materials [3–9].

The field of biomaterials is in continuous growth due to the aging population as well as general population growth. In an effort to regain form and function and increase the quality and duration of human life, biomaterials, which can be artificial or natural, are utilized to repair or replace a biological component that has been lost or destroyed. Biomaterials are employed in many different sections of the human body, including the heart, blood arteries, orthopedic implants, teeth, and stents [2, 10, 11]. They are also used as cardiac pacemakers and for urinary and digestive tract reconstructions. Of all, the largest number of implants is for orthopedic prostheses, such as those for the limbs, spine, hip and knee. According to the current growth in the demand for orthopedic implants, it doubles at least every 10 years, and the demand for knee prostheses triples. This is due to the degenerative illnesses that affect human joints, such as osteoarthritis (joint inflammation), osteoporosis (bone thinning), and trauma, which can cause pain or function loss. Due to excessive stress or the lack of the normal biological self-healing mechanism, degenerative illnesses cause the mechanical characteristics of the bone to deteriorate. Artificial biomaterials are the answers to these issues, and their surgical implantation aids in the functional restoration of structures that might otherwise be impaired. However, revision procedures for hip and knee implants have also grown, in addition to replacement surgery. These painful revision procedures are incredibly costly, and they also have a very poor success rate [2–7].

The goal of current research is to create implants that can last far longer, maybe without failing, and even without the need for revision surgery. Therefore, it is crucial to design a suitable material with a long lifespan, great corrosion resistance in the body environment, a good mix of high strength and low Young's modulus, high fatigue and wear resistance, high ductility, excellent biocompatibility, and no cytotoxicity [1].

Metallic biomaterials, which are typically utilized for support applications, need to have enough fatigue strength to endure the rigors of everyday activity. For applications like articular surfaces in joints and teeth, as well as bone bonding surfaces in implants, ceramic biomaterials are typically chosen for hardness and wear resistance. Polymeric materials have historically been employed for low-friction articulated surfaces due to their flexibility and stability. As a result, titanium becomes one of the most attractive engineering materials for several applications, and due to their exceptional qualities, in its biocompatibility, low modulus and corrosion resistance [5–7, 12–14]. Implant materials should not be harmful and should not result in allergic or inflammatory responses in people. The effectiveness of biomaterials is largely determined by how the body responds to the implant, and this determines a material's biocompatibility. The host reaction a material induces and the degradation of the substance in the bodily environment are the two key determinants of a material's biocompatibility.

The host and implant material respond in a variety of ways when exposed to human tissues and bodily fluids, and these interactions determine whether the implant material is acceptable to the human body.

Issues related to biocompatibility encompass thrombosis, which involves the clotting of blood and the adherence of blood platelets to the surface of biomaterials, as well as the formation of fibrous tissue around implanted biomaterials in soft tissues.

2. Necessary properties of biomaterials

A biomaterial's entry into a living thing impacts how the implant and tissue interact, which might lead to opposing responses. They could be biological, mechanical, electrochemical, or toxicity. Even the utilized assembly or the nearby bone or tissue may sustain severe injury. These occurrences lead to corrosion on the surface of the implant, which degrades its quality depending on the quality of the biomaterial, the location of implantation, and other factors. A biomaterial must have one or more of the following characteristics, depending on the medical application to which it lends itself [15–25].

2.1 Mechanical properties

The selection of a material type is influenced by crucial mechanical properties such as hardness, tensile strength, Young's modulus, and elongation. Biomechanical incompatibility arises when an implant fractures due to mechanical failure. Consequently, it is expected that the chosen material for bone replacement would possess similar mechanical characteristics. The Young's modulus of bone varies between 4 and 30 GPa [15–26], depending on the type of bone and the direction of measurement.

2.2 Osseointegration

Implant loosening is caused by the implant surface's failure to osseointegrate with the surrounding bone and other tissues as a result of motions [27]. Another crucial element of employing metal alloys in bone applications is osseointegration, which is the capacity to join with bone. For the implant to be safe and functional for the duration of its life, bone fusion with the implant is necessary. It is evident that surface chemical and physical features have a significant impact on implant-surface interactions through altering cell behavior, growth factor production, and osteogenic gene development, despite the fact that surface cellular processes are not well known [5, 15–18].

In certain scenarios, despite achieving initial stability of the implant, the bone may experience retraction or become disconnected from the implant due to various factors [14, 28–30]:

- The implant's reaction with foreign substances, leading to toxic emissions from the implant.
- Bone damage or injury resulting from surgical trauma.
- Imposition of abnormal or nonphysiological conditions on the bone, such as fluid pressures or movement against implant components.
- Modification of mechanical signals that promote bone densification.
- Reduction of stress or protection of the replaced or neighboring bone.

2.3 Corrosion testing

In some measure, all metal implants corrode electrochemically. This is bad because the structural integrity is reduced during the degradation process, and the degradation products may negatively affect the host. Wear and electrochemical dissolution are both causes of metal implant deterioration, however the two are most frequently combined to cause degradation. Both generalized dissolution, which evenly affects the whole surface, and localized regions of a component are involved in the electrochemical corrosion process [14, 30]. The strength of the oxidation/reduction processes that drive corrosion (thermodynamic driving forces) and the physical barriers that regulate the kinetics of corrosion are what determine how much metal implant corrosion occurs. These two factors that affect how biomaterials corrode in real life can be broken down into a variety of factors, including: geometrical parameters (e.g. surface microstructure, oxide structure and composition), mechanical variables (e.g. stress and/or relative motion) and solution variables (e.g. pH, proteins in solution and enzymes) [2].

Because metal alloys come in touch with a particularly harsh environment, such as bodily fluid due to the presence of chloride ions and proteins, corrosion resistance of a surgically implanted alloy is a crucial property. The alloy's metal components are converted to their ionic states during the corrosion process, and the dissolved oxygen is transformed into hydroxide ions. The passive coating that forms on an alloy's surface and the presence of alloying elements have a significant impact on how well an alloy resists corrosion.

2.4 Wear resistance

Because of the heterogeneous lubrication regime, wear always happens in artificial joints. An prosthetic hip joint moves, creating billions of minute particles that are removed by the motions. The joint capsule's tissues are home to these particles, which might cause unfavorable responses from external bodies. Histocytes and large cells phagocytose the discharged particles and produce tissues that resemble granulomas. They interfere with bone resorption, which causes osteolysis, at the level of the layer that separates the implant from the bone. The performance of the device is influenced by the use of different materials for the femoral head and cup. Over time, various material and surface treatment combinations have been employed in the development of endoprostheses to minimize wear. Currently, the primary metallic materials utilized for biomedical applications include 316L stainless steel, cobalt chromium alloys (CoCr-), titanium-based alloys (such as Ti-6Al-4V, TiMo-), as well as other materials like tantalum, gold, and dental amalgams. Titanium alloys are increasingly preferred over other materials due to their exceptional qualities, including high strength, low density, excellent corrosion resistance, complete inertness in the body environment, improved compatibility, low Young's modulus, and the ability to fuse with bones or other tissues. These alloys outperform traditional stainless steels and cobalt-based alloys due to their lower Young's modulus, enhanced biocompatibility, and superior corrosion resistance [15–26]. Consequently, titanium and titanium alloys are commonly employed as replacements for hard tissues in artificial bones, joints, and dental implants, given their aforementioned attributes.

2.5 Biocompatibility

One of the most important properties of biomaterials is biocompatibility, which refers to the ability of a material to perform its intended function without causing adverse reactions in the body. The biomaterial should not elicit toxic or immune responses and should be well-tolerated by the host tissue.

2.6 Bioactivity

Biomaterials may have inherent bioactivity, meaning they can interact with the surrounding biological environment to facilitate specific biological responses. For example, bioactive materials can promote cell adhesion, proliferation, and differentiation to support tissue regeneration.

3. Titanium and its alloys

William Gregor initially found titanium as a metal in 1791, but Klaproth gave it the name titanium in 1795. Titanium and its alloys are used in a variety of fields including shipbuilding, aviation, automotive, energy, medicine, and sports equipment due to their low density, high strength-to-weight ratio, good biocompatibility, improved corrosion resistance, plasticity, and good mechanical properties.

Titanium and its alloys are extensively used as biomaterials due to their exceptional biocompatibility, remarkable corrosion resistance, and favorable mechanical properties. These metals possess a specific elastic modulus and low density, which enables them to exhibit mechanical behavior similar to that of bones. Among the materials suitable for implantation in the human body, titanium stands out as it is lightweight, durable, and biocompatible. In the field of biomedicine, commercial pure titanium (C.P. Ti) and its alloys, such as Ti-6Al-4 V and Ti-Mo, are widely employed. They serve as popular alternatives for hard tissue in artificial joints, bones, and dental implants. The low elastic modulus of titanium and its alloys is often considered advantageous in terms of biomechanics, as it can lead to reduced stress shielding [3–7]. Another noteworthy characteristic of titanium-based materials is their tendency to form an extremely thin, adherent, and protective coating of titanium oxide. This feature further enhances the potential of titanium and its alloys as promising biomaterials for implants. One of the main requirements for titanium and its alloys' exceptional biocompatibility and corrosion resistance is the existence of this spontaneously generated oxide coating during the passivation or repassivation process.

Due of its poor mechanical qualities, cp titanium (purely commercial) is used mostly for dental implants in terms of medical applications. Alloys with Al, V, Mo, and other elements are utilized in applications where good mechanical properties are necessary, such as hip implants, knee implants, bone screws, and plates. Artificial hip joints, which comprise of an articulated bearing (femoral head and cup) and stem, are one of the most prevalent uses for titanium alloys. The metal parts of the hip cup and stem are constructed of titanium. They frequently protect the knee joint and have a polyethylene joint surface and titanium femoral and tibial components [3–7].

By adding alloying elements, it gives titanium a wide field of applicability through different microstructure and properties. Thus, the alloying elements are divided into three categories:

- stabilizers α: C, N_2, O_2, Al;
- β stabilizers: V, Nb, Mo, Ta, Fe, Mn, Cr, Co, W, Ni, Cu, Si, H_2;
- neutral elements: Zr, Sn, Hf, Ge, Th.

In the medical field, the Ti-Al-Mo, Ti-Al-Cr, Ti-Al-V, Ti-Al-Cr-Mo systems are used, with excellent biocompatibility in contact with living tissues. Titanium grade 4JSO 5832/11 is used for the manufacture of dental implants. The advantages of using titanium in implantology reside in resistance, reliable technological process of obtaining, easy processing by conventional and non-conventional means, acceptable price.

3.1 Beta-type titanium alloys

Beta-type titanium alloys primarily contain high concentrations of beta-phase stabilizers, giving these alloys a predominantly beta structure at room temperature. While pure titanium has a hexagonal close-packed (hcp) crystal structure, beta-type alloys can contain beta phases with a body-centered cubic structure, providing a unique combination of mechanical and chemical properties.

Some characteristics of beta-type titanium alloys include:

- *High strength*: these alloys can exhibit superior mechanical strength, making them suitable for high-demand applications such as in the aerospace industry or military components.
- *Corrosion resistance*: titanium itself is already corrosion-resistant, but beta-type alloys can enhance this property, making them ideal for use in aggressive environments, such as in the oil and maritime industries.
- *Biocompatibility*: beta-type titanium alloys are known for their high biocompatibility, which means they can be used in medical applications, such as orthopedic or dental implants.
- *Ductility and formability*: these alloys can be processed to obtain a variety of complex shapes due to their ductility.
- *High operating temperature*: some beta-type alloys can be used in applications that require performance at high temperatures.
- *High strength-to-weight ratio*: due to the lightweight nature of titanium and the good mechanical properties of beta-type alloys, these materials have an impressive strength-to-weight ratio, making them ideal for aerospace and space applications.

It is important to mention that the specific properties of a beta-type titanium alloy may vary depending on its exact chemical composition and the manufacturing processes used. By adjusting the proportions of alloying elements, titanium alloys with specific properties can be obtained for various industrial/medical applications.

3.2 Applications of titanium and its alloys

Titanium and its alloys have found extensive applications in various fields due to their unique combination of properties. Here are some few examples of the diverse applications of titanium and its alloys. The unique properties of titanium make it a valuable material in various industries where high strength, corrosion resistance, biocompatibility, and lightweight characteristics are essential.

Biomedical implants: titanium and its alloys are widely used in the field of biomedical implants, such as orthopedic implants (hip and knee replacements, bone plates, and screws), dental implants, and cardiovascular implants. Their biocompatibility, corrosion resistance, and high strength-to-weight ratio make them suitable for long-term implantation in the human body.

Aerospace industry: titanium alloys are extensively utilized in the aerospace industry due to their exceptional strength, lightweight nature, and high heat resistance. They are used in aircraft components, including structural components, landing gear, engine parts, and fasteners, where strength and corrosion resistance are critical.

Chemical processing: titanium and its alloys are resistant to corrosion in various aggressive chemical environments, making them suitable for chemical processing equipment. They are used in reactors, heat exchangers, pipes, valves, and other components that come into contact with corrosive substances.

Marine industry: the excellent corrosion resistance of titanium and its alloys makes them valuable for marine applications. They are used in ship hulls, propellers, offshore structures, and desalination plants, where exposure to seawater and harsh marine environments is prevalent.

Sports equipment: titanium and titanium alloys are employed in sports equipment, particularly in the production of bicycles, golf clubs, tennis rackets, and other lightweight and high-performance sporting goods. The strength, durability, and lightness of titanium contribute to improved performance and reduced weight.

Automotive industry: titanium alloys find limited use in the automotive industry, primarily in high-performance vehicles. They are utilized in exhaust systems, engine components, suspension systems, and other parts where high strength and corrosion resistance are required.

Architecture and design: titanium is increasingly being used in architectural applications due to its esthetic appeal, durability, and resistance to corrosion. It is utilized in building facades, roofs, sculptures, and other artistic structures.

Electronics and consumer goods: titanium and its alloys are utilized in the production of electronic devices and consumer goods. They are employed in smartphones, laptops, watches, jewelry, eyewear frames, and other products where lightweight, corrosion resistance, and esthetic qualities are desired.

4. Novel titanium alloys

Titanium alloys have gained significant popularity and are widely preferred for orthopedic implants in the biomedical field.

In recent years, our research group has focused on obtaining and characterizing new titanium-based alloy recipes with non-toxic elements. This chapter contains a copy of our latest research.

In the study, a series of new recipes were taken, thus several elements were selected such as: Mo, Zr, Ta and Si, to create a β-type titanium alloy. In **Table 1** is presented two main groups of alloys have been developed TMZT (Ti-Mo-Zr-Ta) and TMS (Ti-Mo-Si) with low elastic modulus, strength and good biocompatibility. The titanium alloys were developed in a vacuum electric arc furnace using high purity metals: Ti 99.80%, Mo 99.70%, Zr 99.20%, Ta 99.50% and Si 99.20%. The samples were remelted consecutively at least five times for homogenization.

Proposed alloy	Abbreviation
Ti20Mo	TM
Ti20Mo0,5Si	TM0.5Si
Ti20Mo0,75Si	TM0.75Si
Ti20Mo1Si	TM1Si
Ti20Mo7Zr15Ta	TMZT
Ti20Mo7Zr15Ta 0,5Si	TMZT0.5Si
Ti20Mo7Zr15Ta 0,75Si	TMZT0.75Si
Ti20Mo7Zr15Ta 1Si	TMZT1Si

Table 1.
Developed Ti-based alloys.

The vacuum electric arc furnace is chosen as the method for obtaining titanium alloys due to its ability to produce high-purity materials by minimizing contamination from impurities in the controlled vacuum environment [15, 20].

Adding silicon to Ti-Mo (TM) and Ti-Mo-Zr-Ta (TMZT) alloys can bring several significant benefits. Silicon is an alloying element with specific properties that can enhance the performance and characteristics of these alloys. Here are some of the advantages of adding silicon to these alloys:

- *Phase stabilization*: silicon can help stabilize the alpha and beta phases of titanium. This can lead to improved crystal structure and mechanical properties of the alloys.

- *Increased strength*: the addition of silicon can contribute to the increased strength of Ti-Mo and Ti-Mo-Zr-Ta alloys. This is important in applications that require strong and durable materials.

- *Improved corrosion resistance*: silicon can enhance the corrosion resistance of these alloys, making them suitable for use in aggressive environments or industrial applications.

- *Enhanced biocompatibility*: the addition of silicon can improve the biocompatibility of titanium alloys. This is essential in medical applications, such as orthopedic implants or other medical devices.

- *Reduced density*: silicon has a lower density than titanium, which can lead to a slight reduction in the density of the alloys. This can be beneficial in applications that require lighter materials.

- *Improved high-temperature behavior*: silicon-containing titanium alloys can exhibit better stability at high temperatures, making them suitable for applications involving high-temperature conditions.

It is essential to mention that the exact proportion of silicon and other alloying elements will influence the specific properties of the alloys. Manufacturing processes and heat treatments can also play a crucial role in developing the final characteristics of the alloys.

In conclusion, adding silicon can bring multiple benefits to Ti-Mo and Ti-Mo-Zr-Ta alloys, enhancing their performance and expanding the range of possible applications. In the rest of the chapter, the Ti-Mo, Ti-Mo-Si, Ti-Mo-Zr-Ta and Ti-Mo-Zr-Ta-Si systems will be abbreviated as TM, TMS, TMZT and TMZTS.

4.1 Methodology

Characterization of biomaterials for medical applications involves a comprehensive assessment of their physical, chemical, mechanical, and biological properties.

The new alloys obtained were characterized by the following important techniques in order to demonstrate biocompatibility:

Chemical composition analysis: determining the chemical composition of biomaterials is essential to ensure the desired properties and performance. Techniques such as energy-dispersive X-ray spectroscopy (EDS) can be used to identify the elemental composition. EDS analysis was carried out using an SEM VEGA II LSH electron microscope (TESCAN Co., Czech Republic) equipped with an EDX BRUKER/ROENTEC Co detector (Germany).

Microstructural analysis: this involves examining the microstructure of biomaterials at various length scales using techniques such as optical microscopy, scanning electron microscopy (SEM). Microstructural analysis provides information about the material's surface morphology, grain structure, porosity, and presence of any defects or impurities. The microscopy images, providing high-resolution visualizations, were acquired using a Zeiss Imager 1 M optical microscope, renowned for its advanced imaging capabilities. The microscope was equipped with specialized light and dark field filters, enabling the observation of samples under different illumination conditions and enhancing the contrast and visibility of various features and structures of interest. To investigate the phases present in the materials, we used a Panalytical X'Pert Pro MPD Diffractometer (Malvern Panalytical, The Netherlands).

Mechanical testing: the indentation test is a common method used for mechanical characterization of biomaterials and other materials. It involves applying a controlled force or load to the surface of the material using an indenter, typically a diamond or a hardened steel ball, and measuring the resulting indentation depth or the load-displacement relationship. These tests provide crucial information about the material's ability to withstand mechanical forces and its suitability for specific applications. Some mechanical properties were determined utilizing a CETR UMT-2 tribometer (Bruker, Campbell CA, USA). The assessment involved applying a force of 5 N across a 4 mm distance. The calculated value was the average of three repetitions, and analysis was conducted using the ViEWER program.

Biocompatibility assessment: biomaterials intended for medical applications must undergo biocompatibility evaluation. This involves in vitro and in vivo tests to assess the material's compatibility with living tissues. Techniques include cell culture studies to evaluate cell adhesion, proliferation, and viability, as well as animal studies to assess tissue response, inflammation, and immune reactions.

In vitro biocompatibility tests were conducted on titanium alloy samples by incubating Albino rabbit fibroblasts with the metallic components, measuring cellular metabolic activity using the MTT assay, and comparing the results with a control group; the cell viability was calculated as a percentage based on absorbance readings, and live cells were stained with calcein-AM for fluorescence microscopy imaging.

In vivo studies were conducted on female sheep to evaluate the integration of titanium alloy fragments implanted in the tibial crest, following surgical procedures and ethical guidelines; radiographs and high-resolution CT scans were used to monitor bone repair and peri-implant tissue microstructure, while histological procedures and immunohistochemical staining provided insights into the tissue response and expression of osteopontin, MMP2, and MMP9.

4.2 Results and discussion

4.2.1 Obtaining

The study on the elaboration of Ti-based alloys suggested using an electric arc furnace under a protective atmosphere to ensure homogeneous alloys without metallic inclusions, utilizing high-purity raw materials and a sequence of operations including vacuum melting, purging, and multiple remelting cycles, followed by the preparation of test specimens through cutting, embedding, grinding, and polishing processes.

4.2.2 Chemical composition

The composition, as detailed in **Table 2** [18], provides a comprehensive overview of the specific elements and their respective proportions present in the material under investigation. This table serves as a valuable reference, offering insights into the alloy's composition and aiding in the understanding of its properties and potential applications in various fields. We mention that EDS is not a quantitative method to determine the elemental composition of alloys.

4.2.3 Microstructural results

In **Figures 1** and **2** the specific structure of the studied alloys can be observed, images obtained by optical microscopy. They have a dendritic structure for TMZT alloys. In TMS alloys, a β-type structure can be observed, with the formation of equiaxial grains of different sizes. Acicular and coarse structures specific to β structures are also present [18].

Alloy	Mo	Si	Zr	Ta	Ti
TM	6.01	—	—	—	to 100%
TM0.5Si	6.03	0.14	—	—	to 100%
TM0.75Si	6.12	0.22	—	—	to 100%
TM1Si	6.05	0.31	—	—	to 100%
TMZT	19.00	—	8.15	14.50	to 100%
TMZT0.5Si	18.50	0.45	7.00	14.80	to 100%
TMZT0.75Si	19.50	0.75	6.85	15.04	to 100%
TMZT1Si	19.83	1.03	6.93	14.98	to 100%

Table 2.
Mass composition of alloys obtained by EDS [15, 20] .

The beta structure with dendrites is a characteristic feature observed in certain titanium-based alloys, particularly those containing β-stabilizing elements such as Mo, Zr, Ta, and Si. The beta structure refers to the body-centered cubic (BCC) crystal structure of the beta phase in titanium alloys.

During the solidification process, when the alloy undergoes cooling and transforms from a liquid to a solid state, dendritic growth can occur. Dendrites are tree-like, branching crystal structures that form as a result of anisotropic growth kinetics. In the case of titanium alloys, dendritic growth is commonly observed in the beta phase.

The dendritic structure in the beta phase is formed due to the preferred crystallographic growth directions, resulting in the elongated and branched morphology of the grains. The dendritic branches extend into the surrounding matrix, creating a complex network of interconnected structures. This dendritic morphology provides an increased surface area, allowing for more efficient diffusion and solid-state transformations within the material.

The presence of dendrites in the beta phase affects the microstructure of the alloy. The dendritic structure influences various properties of the material, including mechanical strength, thermal stability, and phase transformation behavior. The size, shape, and distribution of dendrites can be controlled through different processing techniques, such as adjusting the cooling rate during solidification or employing grain refiners.

Furthermore, the dendritic structure in the beta phase can have an impact on the macroscopic properties of the alloy. For example, the alignment and connectivity of dendrites can influence the anisotropy of mechanical properties, such as yield

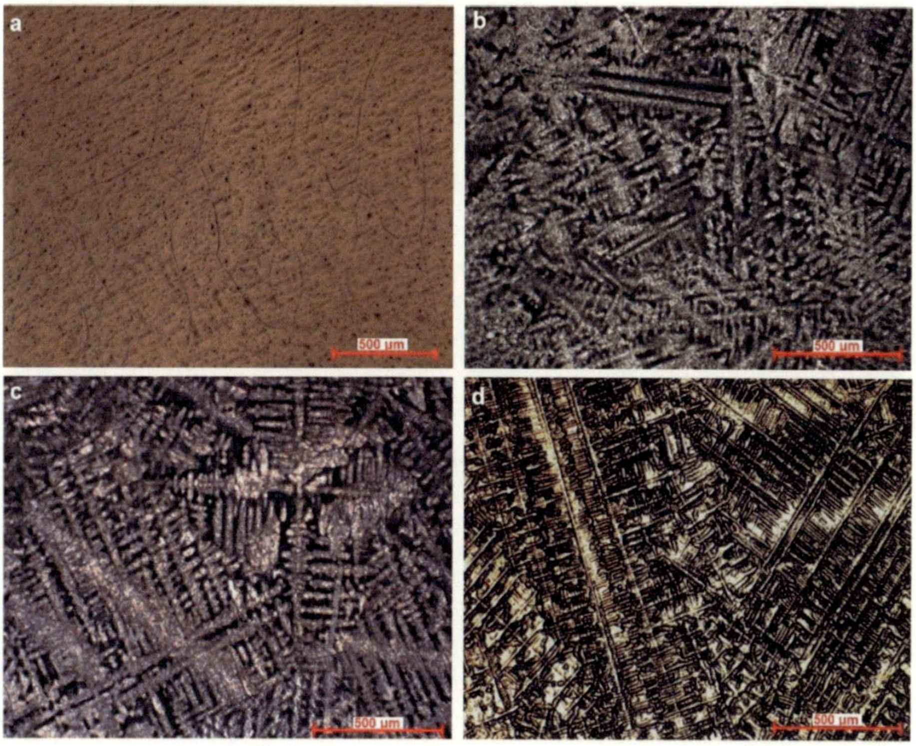

Figure 1.
Optical microstructure of the alloys at 100X. (a) TM, (b) TM0.5Si, (c) TM0.75Si, and (d) TM1Si [17].

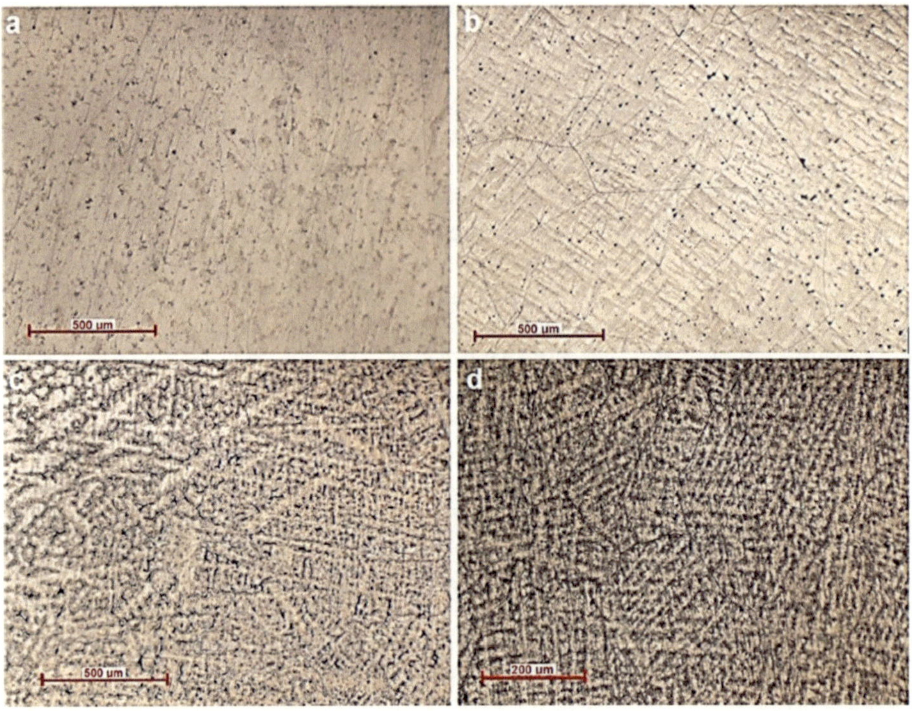

Figure 2.
Optical microscopy images (a) TMZT, (b) TMZT0.5Si, (c) TMZT0.75Si, and (d) TMZT1Si [15].

strength and fracture toughness. The interconnected dendritic network can also affect the diffusion paths and the kinetics of phase transformations, leading to changes in the alloy's thermal and chemical stability.

Based on the study of Ti-based alloys, including TMS and TMZTS systems, it can be concluded that the microstructure of these alloys is strongly influenced by the elaboration method employed.

Based on the diffractograms of the TM*x*Si (x = 0, 0.5, 0.75, 1 wt.%) TMZT*x*Si alloys (x = 0, 0.5, 0.75, 1 wt.%), it can be concluded that the alloys exhibit a predominantly face-centered cubic (fcc) structure (**Figure 3**). The primary phase present in these alloys is the β phase, which is characterized by a centered volume cubic structure. However, there are also minor secondary phases observed, including the α0 martensite phase and the α phase.

The β phase in the diffractograms of Ti-based alloys refers to a specific crystallographic phase known as the beta phase. This phase is characterized by a centered volume cubic structure and is commonly present in Ti alloys. The diffractograms indicate the presence and relative abundance of the β phase in the analyzed TMZTS alloys.

The β phase is an important constituent in Ti alloys as it significantly influences their mechanical properties, such as strength and ductility. It is a solid solution phase that can accommodate various alloying elements, including Mo, Zr, Ta, and Si, depending on the specific alloy composition. The presence of these alloying elements can modify the lattice parameters and stabilize the β phase, leading to improved mechanical performance.

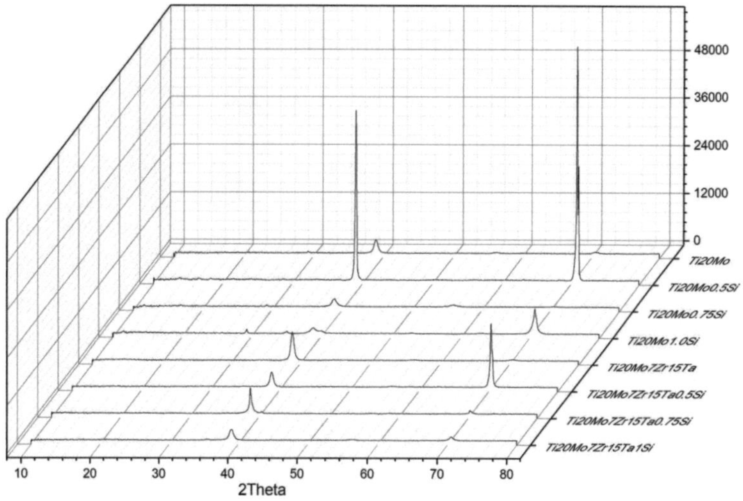

Figure 3.
Diffractograms alloys studied [15, 17, 20].

In the diffractograms, the peaks corresponding to the β phase can be identified and analyzed to determine the crystallographic orientation and phase purity. The positions and intensities of these peaks provide information about the arrangement of atoms within the crystal lattice and the presence of any additional phases.

The diffractograms may also reveal the presence of minor secondary phases, such as the α0 martensite phase and the α phase. These secondary phases can form due to the decomposition of the β phase during the cooling process or as a result of specific alloy compositions. Their presence can affect the overall microstructure and mechanical behavior of the Ti-based alloys.

By analyzing the diffractograms, researchers can gain insights into the crystalline structure, phase composition, and phase transformations occurring in TMZTS alloys. This information is valuable for understanding the alloy's properties and optimizing its performance for various applications, such as aerospace, biomedical implants, and structural materials.

4.2.4 Mechanical properties

In **Table 3** are presented the specific mechanical properties obtained through indentation for each alloy within the TMS and TMZT systems, highlighting their respective Young's modulus, hardness, and specimen Poisson Ratio. This analysis will provide valuable insights into the mechanical behavior and potential applications of these alloys, aiding in the advancement of materials science and engineering.

The comparison reveals how different alloy compositions within each system impact the mechanical properties. Additionally, the comparison between the TMS and TMZT systems provides valuable information on the influence of alloying elements on the overall material characteristics. **Figure 4** shows a graphic comparison of the modulus of elasticity between the classic alloys and the newly developed titanium alloys. As can be seen, the newly developed alloys have a very low modulus of elasticity compared to classic alloys.

Alloy	Young modulus (GPa)	Hardness (HV)	Specimen Poisson Ration
TM	57.54	376.30	0.23
TM0.5Si	37.86	239.60	0.23
TM0.75Si	29.06	216.20	0.23
TM1Si	26.22	210.80	0.23
TMZT	53.58	305.34	0.23
TMZT0.5Si	54.25	339.24	0.23
TMZT0.75Si	56.38	315.27	0.23
TMZT1Si	63.88	274.64	0.23

Table 3.
Some mechanical characteristics of alloys obtained by indentation [15, 20].

The TMZT system generally displays higher Young's modulus and hardness values compared to the TMS system. This implies that the TMZT system alloys possess greater stiffness and better resistance to wear and deformation. However, it's important to note that the specific alloy compositions and intended applications can further influence the performance and suitability of these systems.

In orthopedics, the Young's modulus is of paramount importance as it directly influences the performance and behavior of implant materials used in prosthetic devices, joint replacements, and other orthopedic applications. A suitable Young's modulus is crucial to ensure that the implant material closely matches the mechanical properties of the surrounding natural tissues. If the implant's Young's modulus is significantly different from that of the bone or tissue, it may cause stress concentrations, leading to potential implant failure, discomfort, or long-term complications.

Comparing Ti-based alloys to classical alloys used in orthopedics, such as stainless steels or cobalt-chromium alloys, the Ti-based alloys obtained exhibit a lower Young's modulus. This lower modulus makes Ti-based alloys more favorable for orthopedic implants since they are closer in mechanical properties to natural bone. By mimicking the elasticity of bone, Ti-based alloys can help reduce the stress shielding effect that occurs when a stiffer implant causes bone resorption due to inadequate load transfer to the surrounding bone. Consequently, Ti-based alloys have the advantage of potentially providing a more successful and long-lasting integration with the patient's bone, improving the overall performance and biocompatibility of orthopedic implants.

Overall, these alloys exhibit a range of mechanical characteristics, such as stiffness, hardness, and consistent response to applied forces. Each alloy's unique combination of properties makes them suitable for specific applications, allowing for versatility and tailored performance in various engineering scenarios.

4.2.5 In vitro studies

Biocompatibility in vitro is of paramount importance in the evaluation and development of biomedical materials and implants. It involves studying the interactions between the materials and living cells under controlled laboratory conditions. The importance of in vitro biocompatibility testing lies in its ability to provide valuable insights into the potential effects of materials on cellular behavior, viability, and functionality.

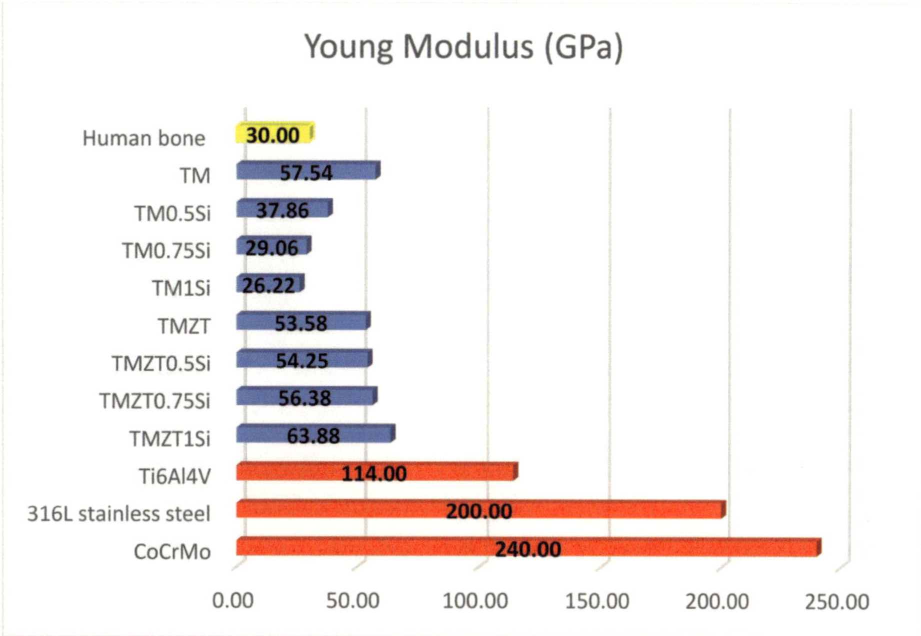

Figure 4.
Graphical comparison of the modulus of elasticity.

By subjecting materials to cell cultures, researchers can evaluate factors such as cell adhesion, proliferation, metabolic activity, and morphology. These assessments help determine the compatibility of the materials with living tissues and cells, providing essential information for biomedical applications. Furthermore, in vitro biocompatibility testing allows for the identification of potential cytotoxic effects or adverse reactions that may arise from the interaction between materials and cells.

In the case of the presented study, primary Albino rabbit fibroblasts were utilized to assess the biocompatibility of the alloys. The use of standardized protocols and tests such as the MTT assay ensures reliable and reproducible data, allowing for accurate comparisons between different materials and controls.

Understanding the biocompatibility of materials is crucial for the development of safe and effective biomedical devices, implants, and drug delivery systems. In vitro testing serves as an initial step in the evaluation process, providing valuable information before progressing to more complex in vivo and clinical studies.

Experimental procedures:

- The biocompatibility of the alloys was assessed through in vitro tests using primary Albino rabbit fibroblasts.
- Cellular metabolic activity was measured using the 3-(4,5-dimethylthiazol-2-yl)-2,5-diphenyltetrazolium bromide (MTT) assay, and the results were compared with a control group [20, 30–33].
- A solution called penicillin/streptomycin/neomycin (P/S/N), composed of specific quantities of penicillin, streptomycin, and neomycin in sterile water,

was used as the standard modified Dulbecco's Eagle medium (DMEM) for cell culture [34–37].

- The experimental procedure involved seeding cells in 12-well plates at an initial density of 5×10^3 cells/cm^2 in complete medium and incubating them overnight at 37°C and 5% CO_2.

- The alloy samples were disinfected using a sterile 70% ethyl alcohol solution for 30 min, followed by washing with sterile water and phosphate-buffered saline (PBS) [34–37].

- Decontaminated samples were then placed in DMEM complete culture media and cultured for 24 h at 37°C, 5% CO_2, and 97% humidity.

- The pre-plated cells received the sterilized alloy samples and were cultured for different time intervals (24, 48, and 72 h).

- MTT assays were performed at each time point to assess cell viability.

- After the incubation, MTT working solution was added to the cells and incubated in the dark at 37°C and 97% humidity.

- The formation of MTT formazan crystals, indicative of live cells, was observed and dissolved using acidified isopropanol.

- The colored solution was measured at a wavelength of 570 nm using a Tecan plate reader modified with Magellan V7.1SP1 Sunrise model software.

- Cell viability was calculated as a percentage using absorbance values, comparing cells cultured with the metal alloys to the control group incubated with PBS [20].

- Additionally, live cells were stained with calcein-AM, a fluorescent dye that produces green fluorescence in live cells.

- Albino rabbit fibroblasts and the human osteosarcoma cell line MG63 were employed for this staining.

- The cell-populated metal alloys were washed with HBSS and stained with calcein-AM according to the kit's instructions.

- The hydrolyzed calcein fluorescence was visualized using a fluorescence microscope with a 455 nm excitation and 530 nm emission filter [20].

In conclusions, the cytocompatibility assessment of the metallic materials was successfully conducted using in vitro tests with cell cultures. Primary Albino rabbit fibroblasts were chosen as the cell model for these experiments. The evaluation of cell viability was performed through the MTT test, which involved incubating the metal alloys with cell cultures for varying durations (24, 48, and 72 h). These assessments provided valuable insights into the biocompatibility of the alloys and their potential for biomedical applications.

Figures 5 and **6** present the data obtained from the MTT assay, showing the calculated cell viabilities for the different alloys at each time point. These figures provide a visual representation of the cytocompatibility of the alloys and allow for a direct comparison with the control group.

The results of the cytocompatibility tests for both TMS and TMZTS systems revealed promising outcomes. According to the ISO 10933-5 standards, all tested TMZTS alloys demonstrated cytocompatibility, as shown in **Figures 5** and **6**. This indicates that these alloys have the potential to interact favorably with biological systems without causing harmful effects.

The calculated cell viability for all examined materials surpassed the threshold of 85%, which is a significant indicator of their biocompatibility. This suggests that the cells were able to maintain their metabolic activity and proliferate effectively in the presence of the alloys. The high cell viability further supports the notion that these materials have the potential to be used in biomedical applications.

Interestingly, the addition of silicon to the alloys did not have any discernible impact on the vitality of the fibroblasts. This implies that the incorporation of silicon did not compromise the biocompatibility of the alloys and suggests that Si can be effectively incorporated into these systems without compromising their cytocompatibility.

These findings are consistent with earlier investigations cited in the references [20, 38–42]. The alignment of these results with previous studies reinforces the reliability and validity of the current findings, adding to the body of knowledge supporting the cytocompatibility of TMZTS alloys. Collectively, these results provide strong evidence that the TMZTS alloys have excellent biocompatibility, making them suitable candidates for various biomedical applications.

After 72 h of cell culture involving primary albino rabbit fibroblast cells and the human osteosarcoma cell line MG63, the fibroblasts were extracted from the alloy samples and their morphology was examined using phase contrast and fluorescence optical microscopy. **Figure 7** illustrate the final photographs obtained from this analysis.

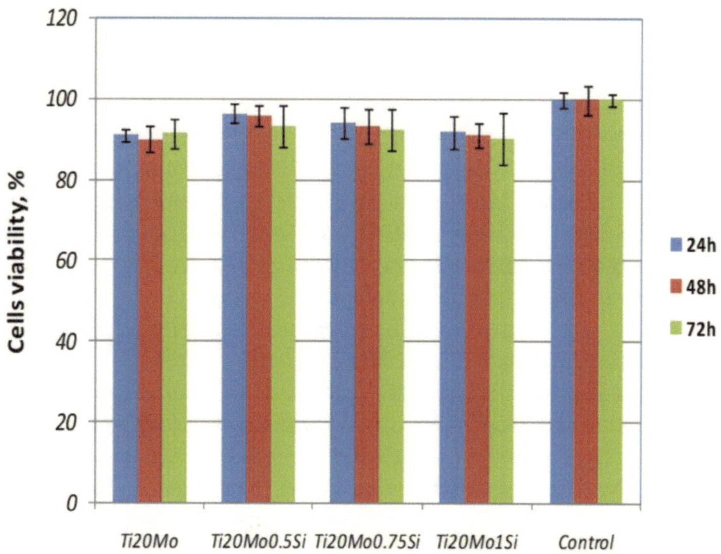

Figure 5.
Mitochondrial activity measured via the MTT assessment for TMS group [20].

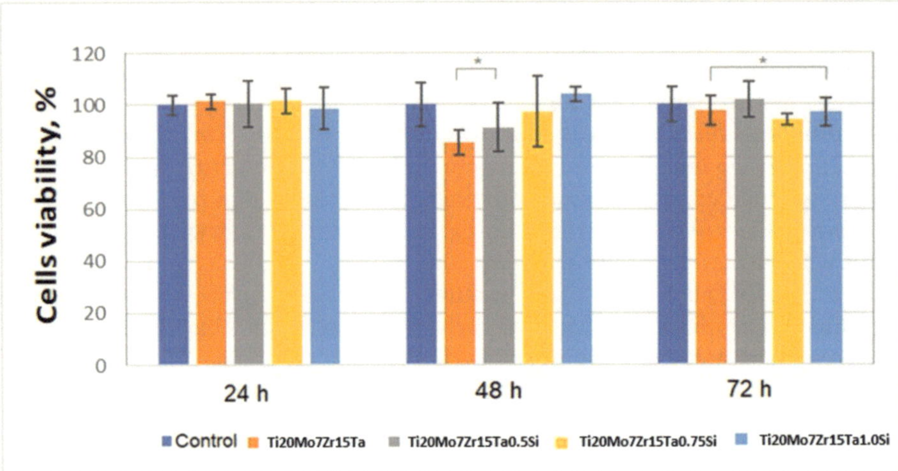

Figure 6.
Mitochondrial activity measured via the MTT assessment for TMZTS group [15].

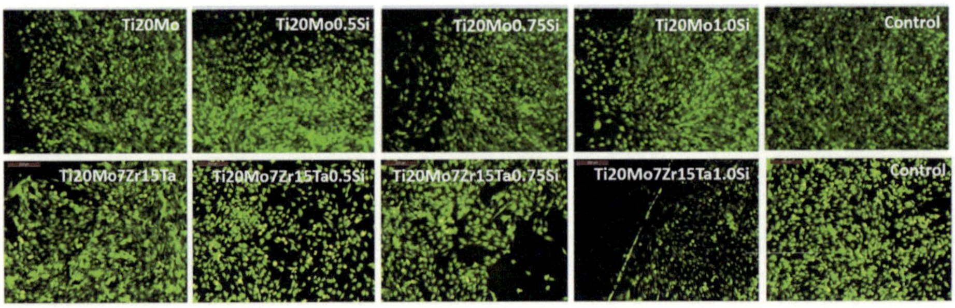

Figure 7.
Fluorescent microscopy (calcein AM) results for TMZTS alloys in contact with cell cultures for 72 h [15, 20].

The microscopy observations revealed that the cells formed a monolayer in direct contact with the alloy samples, which appeared as dark areas in the images. Interestingly, there were no significant differences observed in comparison to the growth of the control sample. The cells displayed elongated shapes with a fibroblastic morphology, while the osteoblasts appeared smaller and more spherical. The presence of dark regions in the images could be attributed to the positioning of substances, indicating that the material might generate mechanical activities that potentially compromise the integrity of the cell monolayer.

Regarding cell growth density, the line osteoblasts exhibited a higher density compared to primary fibroblasts. This difference can be attributed to the behavior of the line cells, specifically MG63 osteoblasts, which have a faster growth rate compared to the more sensitive primary cells [20, 39–42]. However, a comprehensive analysis of the microscope data for both types of cultures demonstrates that the TMS and TMZTS alloys do not have any discernible effect on cell shape or growth. Both the fibroblast and osteoblast cells displayed comparable appearances to the growth control, indicating a high level of cytocompatibility [20, 39–42].

The microscopy analysis provides strong evidence supporting the cytocompatibility of the TMS and TMZTS alloys. The cells maintained their normal growth patterns and shapes when in contact with the alloy surfaces, reinforcing the potential of these alloys for various biomedical applications where maintaining cell viability and morphology is necessary.

4.2.6 In vivo studies

In vivo studies are of great importance as they provide crucial insights into the behavior and performance of materials or interventions within living organisms, allowing for a more comprehensive evaluation of their safety, efficacy, and compatibility. These studies bridge the gap between in vitro experiments and clinical applications, providing valuable information on biological responses, tissue interactions, and potential adverse effects in a complex physiological environment. By simulating real-life conditions, in vivo studies play a pivotal role in guiding the development, optimization, and translation of new materials, treatments, and medical devices, ultimately enhancing patient outcomes and ensuring the highest standards of biomedical research.

For in vivo study, TMS alloys were implanted into the tibial crest of four adult female sheep (one control and three experimental), following a surgical procedure and strict adherence to ethical guidelines and regulations (**Figure 8**). And the TMZTS alloys were implanted 60-day on five rabbits (Orychtolagus cuniculus) of both genders (**Figure 9**).

Experiments on the TMS system reconfirmed the use of Ti-based alloys, known as bioinert biomaterials, in the implantation process induces contact and distance osteogenesis through an interference bond with the surrounding tissue. The blood parameters of the control and experimental sheep remained stable throughout the experiment, indicating no significant changes. The spontaneously formed titanium oxide layer proved to be highly stable, effectively separating the alloy from neighboring tissues. X-ray and CT evaluations demonstrated the presence of a clear space surrounding each implant, bordered by fibrous-cartilaginous tissue, without any local abnormal bone reactions.

In the control sheep, moderate physiological osteolysis was observed in the area of the entrance channel, filled with newly formed low-density tissue. The titanium alloys (TM and TM0.5Si) exhibited a greater amount of connective tissue separating them from the bone tissue, with no local reactions. However, the TM0.75Si alloy showed a faster binding to the surrounding tissue, as confirmed by histological examination.

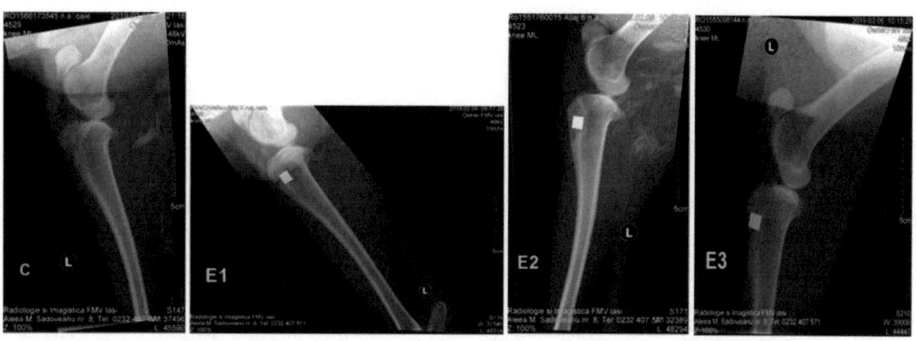

Figure 8.
X-ray images from the control (C) and experimental sheep (E1–E3) for TMS alloys at the 62 days of experiment [20].

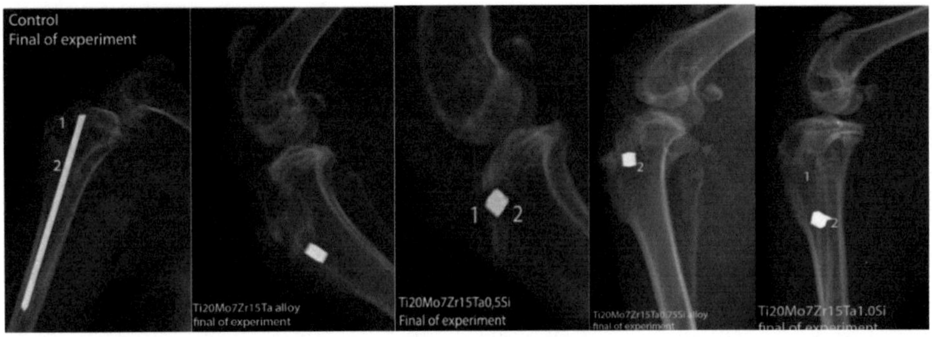

Figure 9.
X-rays of control and experimental rabbits after 60 days of experiment for TMZTS alloys [15].

The presence of molybdenum and silicon in the alloys contributed to their excellent stability and compatibility, comparable to pure titanium.

Histological analysis revealed periosteum proliferation and ossification following a membranous model in the experimental groups, while a mixture of membranous, enchondral, and membranous ossification was observed in the control sheep. The connective tissue near the bone breach exhibited rich vascularity, and the capsules surrounding the implants were thick and poorly vascularized. The connective tissue contained osteoprogenitor cells and newly formed bone tissue. Bone trabeculae alternated between mineralized and non-mineralized areas. Mesenchymal stem cells differentiated into osteoblasts, actively contributing to bone formation.

Immunohistochemical analysis demonstrated the presence of osteopontin (OSP) in cells, indicating intense activity of osteoprogenitor cells involved in matrix mineralization and osteoblasts in the areolae. MMP2 and MMP9 expression was observed in the interface matrix between the implant and the bone remodeling area. MMP2 was particularly present in osteocytes, involved in solubilizing the osteoid. MMP9 played a role in controlling osteoclast maturation and migration, with expression observed in mesenchymal stem cells, osteoblasts, osteocytes, and giant multinucleated cells.

For TMZTS system, the X-ray investigations conducted on experimental rabbits after 60 days of the experiment revealed no abnormal radiological changes in both the control and implanted rabbits. The radiodensity of the peri-implant tissues varied depending on the alloy used, with values ranging from 300 to 931 Hounsfield Units (HU) for peri-implanted tissues in control and implanted rabbits. The newly formed tissue in the implantation gap exhibited a radiopacity of about 793 HU, while the radio-opacity in the peri-implant area ranged from 633 to 931 HU for TMZT1Si alloy and 400–651 HU for TMZT alloy.

Histological analyses confirmed the presence of fibrous intramembranous ossification tissues associated with the radiopacity observed in the newly formed tissues around the implants. Different alloys showed varying degrees of osteogenesis, with TMZT0.75Si and TMZT0.5Si alloys exhibiting mesenchymal cells in the fibrous capsule and newly formed bone tissue containing a small number of bone lamellae. TMZTS alloy demonstrated both intramembranous and endochondral types of ossification.

Osteopontin (OPN) expression was observed in all experimental groups, with an overexpression observed in the bone interface area for TMZT0.5Si, TMZT0.75Si, and TMZTS groups. Metalloproteinases (MMPs), specifically MMP2 and MMP9, also showed overexpression in all experimental groups, indicating their involvement in the cellular and physiological processes of bone formation, tissue repair, angiogenesis, and morphogenesis.

As a conclusion, the findings suggest that the implanted alloys triggered osteogenesis and healing processes, leading to the formation of new bone tissue. The presence of OPN and MMPs further supports the role of these molecules in bone remodeling and regeneration.

From an in vitro point of view, both the TMS and TMZTS systems have shown promising results in terms of their biocompatibility and potential for bone regeneration.

The TMS system demonstrated good cell viability and proliferation, indicating its compatibility with living cells. The addition of silicon to the alloy composition promoted the formation of a biocompatible oxide layer on the surface, which could enhance osseointegration. Furthermore, the TMS system exhibited favorable mechanical properties, such as adequate strength and elastic modulus, making it suitable for load-bearing applications.

Similarly, the TMZTS system exhibited good cytocompatibility, supporting cell attachment, proliferation, and spreading. The incorporation of zirconium and tantalum in the alloy composition provided enhanced mechanical properties, including increased strength and corrosion resistance. The addition of silicon further improved the biocompatibility and potential for bone tissue integration.

Both systems showed the formation of new bone tissue around the implants, as indicated by the histological analyses. The presence of fibrous intramembranous ossification tissues and the expression of osteopontin and metalloproteinases suggested active bone formation and remodeling processes [43, 44].

Overall, the TMS and TMZTS systems demonstrated promising in vitro biocompatibility, mechanical properties, and ability to support bone regeneration. These findings warrant further investigation and evaluation in in vivo studies to assess their long-term performance and potential for clinical applications.

5. Conclusions

In conclusion, the TMS and TMZTS systems have shown promising results across various aspects, including mechanical properties, biocompatibility, and their ability to support bone regeneration, based on in vitro studies.

From a mechanical perspective, both systems exhibited favorable properties, including adequate strength, corrosion resistance, and elastic modulus. These properties are crucial for implant materials as they ensure stability, longevity, and appropriate load-bearing capacity, which are essential for successful clinical applications.

In terms of biocompatibility, both systems demonstrated good cytocompatibility, supporting cell viability, proliferation, and attachment. This indicates that the alloys are well-tolerated by living cells and have the potential to integrate with surrounding tissues. The presence of fibrous intramembranous ossification tissues and the expression of osteopontin and metalloproteinases further suggest active bone formation and remodeling processes, indicating a positive biological response to the materials.

Additionally, both systems showed the formation of new bone tissue around the implants, indicating their ability to support bone regeneration. This is a crucial factor for implant success, as it allows for the establishment of a strong bond between the implant and the surrounding bone, promoting long-term stability.

However, it is important to note that these conclusions are based on in vitro studies, and further investigation through in vivo studies is necessary to validate and assess the long-term performance of the TMS and TMZTS systems. In vivo studies can provide insights into the materials' behavior within a living organism, including their interaction with the host tissue, potential immune responses, and overall biocompatibility. Only through comprehensive in vivo evaluations can the clinical potential of these systems be fully understood and their suitability for human applications be determined.

6. Future trends

The titanium-based alloys used both in dental prosthetics and orthopedics have special properties, being involved in most interventions involving the replacement of an anatomical tissue or element.

Thus, the growing demand of the market has pushed research in the direction of extending the life of implants, through the development of new biocompatible materials.

Evaluating the results obtained following the full characterization of the alloys, we can conclude that the new systems obtained have a reduced modulus of elasticity, without showing cytotoxicity at the cellular or tissue level.

The obtained systems can be successfully used in various medical applications, such as dental and orthopedic implants.

Acknowledgements

This paper was financially supported by the Project "Network of excellence in applied research and innovation for doctoral and postdoctoral programs/ InoHubDoc", project co-funded by the European Social Fund financing agreement no. POCU/993/6/13/153437. This paper was also supported by "Gheorghe Asachi" Technical University from Iaşi (TUIASI), through the Project "Performance and excellence in postdoctoral research 2022".

Conflict of interest

The authors declare no conflict of interest.

Author details

Petrica Vizureanu[1,2]*, Madalina Simona Baltatu[1] and Andrei Victor Sandu[1,3]

1 Faculty of Materials Science and Engineering, Department of Technologies and Equipments for Materials Processing, "Gheorghe Asachi" Technical University of Iaşi, Iasi, Romania

2 Technical Sciences Academy of Romania, Bucharest, Romania

3 Academy of Romanian Scientists, Bucharest, Romania

*Address all correspondence to: peviz2002@yahoo.com

References

[1] Wang M, Guo L, Sun H. Manufacture of biomaterials. In: Narayan R, editor. Encyclopedia of Biomedical Engineering. The Netherlands: Elsevier; 2019. pp. 116-134

[2] de Viteri VS, Fuentes E. Titanium and Titanium alloys as Biomaterials, in Tribology - Fundamentals and Advancements. London, United Kingdom: IntechOpen; 2013. DOI: 10.5772/55860

[3] Antoniac I, editor. Handbook of Bioceramics and Biocomposites. Switzerland: Springer; 2016

[4] Ghiban B. Metalic Biomaterials. Bucuresti, Romania: Editura Printech; 1999

[5] Baltatu MS, Vizureanu P. Materiale Biocompatibile. Iasi, Romania: Editura PIM; 2019

[6] Vizureanu P, Baltatu MS. Titanium-Based Alloys for Biomedical Applications. Vol. 74. Millersville, USA: Materials Research Forum LLC; 2020

[7] Vizureanu P, Baltatu MS, Sandu AV. Development of new advanced Ti-Mo alloys for medical applications. Biomaterials. 2020:2-16. DOI: 10.5772/intechopen.919062-16

[8] Chen Q, Thouas GA. Metallic implant biomaterials. Materials Science and Engineering. 2015;**R 87**:1-57. DOI: 10.1016/j.mser.2014.10.001

[9] Santavirta S, Gristina A, Konttinen YT. Cemented versus cementless hip arthroplasty: A review of prosthetic biocompatibility. Acta Orthopaedica Scandinavica. 1992;**63**:225-232

[10] Park JB, Bronzino LD, editors. Biomaterials: Principles and Applications. Boca Raton, Florida: CC Press; 2003. pp. 1-241

[11] Wise DL. Biomaterials Engineering and Devices. Berlin: Human Press; 2000

[12] Wang K. The use of titanium for medical applications in the USA. Materials Science and Engineering A. 1996;**213**:134-137

[13] Williams DF. On the mechanisms of biocompatibility. Biomaterials. 2008;**29**(20):1941-2953

[14] Black J, Hastings GW. Handbook of Biomaterials Properties. London, UK: Chapman and Hall; 1998. DOI: 10.5772/55860

[15] Spataru MC, Cojocaru FD, Sandu AV, Solcan C, Duceac IA, Baltatu MS, et al. Assessment of the effects of si addition to a new TiMoZrTa system. Materials. 2021;**14**(24):Article Number 7610. DOI: 10.3390/ma14247610

[16] Baltatu MS, Spataru MC, Verestiuc L, Balan V, Solcan C, Sandu AV, et al. Design, synthesis, and preliminary evaluation for Ti-Mo-Zr-Ta-Si alloys for potential implant applications. Materials. 2021;**14**(22):Article Number 6806. DOI: 10.3390/ma14226806

[17] Baltatu MS, Vizureanu P, Sandu AV, Florido-Suarez N, Saceleanu MV, Mirza-Rosca JC. New titanium alloys, promising materials for medical devices. Materials. 2021;**14**(20):Article Number 5934. DOI: 10.3390/ma14205934

[18] Sandu AV, Baltatu MS, Nabialek M, Savin A, Vizureanu P. Characterization and mechanical proprieties of new TiMo

alloys used for medical applications. Materials. 2019;**12**:art. 2973

[19] Verestiuc L, Spataru MC, Baltatu MS, Butnaru M, Solcan C, Sandu AV, et al. New Ti–Mo–Si materials for bone prosthesis applications. Journal of the Mechanical Behavior of Biomedical Materials. 2021;**113**:104198. DOI: 10.1016/j.jmbbm.2020.104198

[20] Spataru MC, Butnaru M, Sandu AV, Vulpe V, Vlad MD, Baltatu MS, et al. In-depth assessment of new Ti-based biocompatible materials. Materials Chemistry and Physics. 2021;**258**:Article number 123959. DOI: 10.1016/j.matchemphys.2020.123959

[21] Baltatu MS, Vizureanu P, Sandu AV, Munteanu C, Istrate B. Microstructural analysis and tribological behavior of Ti-based alloys with a ceramic layer using the thermal spray method. Coatings. 2020;**10**:1216. DOI: 10.3390/coatings10121216

[22] Baltatu MS, Tugui CA, Perju MC, Benchea M, Spataru MC, Sandu AV, et al. Biocompatible titanium alloys used in medical applications. Revista de Chimie. 2019;**70**(4):1302-1306

[23] Baltatu MS, Sandu AV, Nabialek M, Vizureanu P, Ciobanu G. Biomimetic deposition of hydroxyapatite layer on titanium alloys. Micromachines. 2021;**12**(12):Article Number 1447. DOI: 10.3390/mi12121447

[24] Focsaneanu SC, Vizureanu P, Sandu AV, Ciobanu G, Baltatu SM, Vlad D. Experimental study on the influence of zirconia surface preparation on deposition of hydroxyapatite. Revista de Chimie. 2019;**70**(6):2273-2275

[25] Baltatu MS, Vizureanu P, Cimpoesu R, Abdullah MMAB, Sandu AV. The corrosion behavior of TiMoZrTa alloys used for medical applications. Revista de Chimie. 2016;**67**(10):2100-2102

[26] Lawrence Katz J. Anisotropy of Young's modulus of bone. Nature. 1980;**283**:106-107

[27] Viceconti M, Muccini R, Bernakiewicz M, Baleani M, Cristofolini L. Large-sliding contact elements accurately predict levels of bone-implant micromotion relevant to osseointegration. Journal of Biomechanics. 2000;**33**:1611-1618

[28] Montanaro L, Campoccia D, Arciola CR. Nanostructured materials for inhibition of bacterial adhesion in orthopedic implants: A minireview. International Journal of Artificial Organs. 2008;**31**:771-776

[29] Black J. Othopaedic Biomaterials in Research and Practice. New York: Churchill Livingstone; 1988

[30] Jacobs JJ, Gilbert JL, Urban RM. Corrosion of metal orthopaedic implants. Journal of Bone and Joint Surgery, American. 1998;**80**:268-282

[31] Hwang IJ, Choe HC. Surface morphology and cell behavior of Zn-coated Ti-6Al-4V alloy by RF-sputtering after PEO-treatment. Surface and Coating Technology. 2019;**361**:386-395. DOI: 10.1016/j.surfcoat.2019.01.061

[32] Shahriyari F, Razaghian A, Taghiabadi R, Peirovi A, Amini A. Effect of friction hardening pre-treatment on increasing cytocompatibility of alkali heat-treated Ti-6Al-4V alloy. Surface and Coating Technology. 2018;**353**:148-157

[33] Ozan S, Lin J, Li Y, Wen C. New Ti-Ta-Zr-Nb alloys with ultrahigh

strength for potential orthopedic implant applications. Journal of the Mechanical Behavior of Biomedical Materials. 2017;**75**:119-127

[34] Xu JL, Tao SC, Bao LZ, Luo JM, Zheng YF. Effects of Mo contents on the microstructure, properties and cytocompatibility of the microwave sintered porous Ti-Mo alloys. Materials Science and Engineering C. 2019;**97**:156-165

[35] Czekanska EM, Stoddart MJ, Ralphs JR, Richards RG, Hayes JS. A phenotypic comparison of osteoblast cell lines versus human primary osteoblasts for biomaterials testing. Journal of Biomedical Materials Research A. 2013;**102**:2636-2643

[36] Schwarz F, Langer M, Hagena T, Hartig B, Sader R, Becker J. Cytotoxicity and proinflammatory effects of titanium and zirconia particles. International Journal of Implant Dentistry. 2019;**5**:25. DOI: 10.1186/s40729-019-0178-2

[37] Bodhak S, Bose S, Kinsel WC, Bandyopadhyay A. Investigation of in vitro bone cell adhesion and proliferation on Ti using direct current stimulation. Materials Science and Engineering C. 2012;**32**:2163-2168

[38] Long M, Rack HJ. Titanium alloys in total joint replacement—A materials science perspective. Biomaterials. 1998;**19**:1621-1639

[39] Campoccia D, Montanaro L, Arciola CR. A review of the biomaterials technologies for infection-resistant surfaces. Biomaterials. 2013;**34**:8533-8554

[40] Abdel-Hady Gepreel M, Niinomi M. Biocompatibility of Ti-alloys for long-term implantation. Journal of the Mechanical Behavior of Biomedical Materials. 2013;**20**:407-415

[41] Okada Y, Naka K, Kawamura K, Matsumoto T, Nakanishi I, Fujimoto N, et al. Localization of matrix metalloproteinase-9 (92-kilodalton gelatinase/type IV collagenase = gelatinase B) in osteoclasts: Implications for bone resorption. Laboratory Investigations. 1995;**72**(3):311-322

[42] Suda T, Takahashi N, Udagawa N, Jimi E, Gillespie MT, Martin TJ. Modulation of osteoclast differentiation and function by the new members of the tumor necrosis factor receptor and ligand families. Endocrinology Review. 1999;**20**(3):345-357

[43] Antoniac I, Miculescu M, Mănescu (Păltânea) V, Stere A, Quan PH, Păltânea G, et al. Magnesium-based alloys used in orthopedic surgery. Materials. 2022;**15**:1148

[44] Istrate B, Munteanu C, Antoniac I-V, Lupescu S-C. Current research studies of Mg–Ca–Zn biodegradable alloys used as orthopedic implants—Review. Crystals. 2022;**12**:1468

Section 2

Trends on Tissue Engineering

Chapter 6

Nanofibers for Skin Regeneration and Wound Dressing Applications

Farida ElGamal

Abstract

The regeneration of skin because of numerous sorts of injuries such as burns, wounds, tissue damage, and eczema is regarded as vital; nevertheless, the process of healing and remodeling can be impeded by several reasons. The cutting-edge of nanofibrous technology offers the opportunity to repurpose and innovate new therapies and improve the effectiveness of the available medical treatments. There may be less need for skin transplants and skin grafts as regenerative medicine advances using biopolymeric materials. Skin injuries can be difficult to treat, especially when it comes to managing wounds. The fabrication of different dosage forms such as film, foam, sponge, hydrogel, and nanofiber membranes using scaffolding material made from synthetic and natural polymers is considered a treatment method for wounds. Scaffolds have found applicability in tissue engineering, where the materials are fabricated into artificial tissue that stimulates growth factors and enhances tissue regeneration. Among these materials, nanofibers possess a unique structure of small pore size and high porosity, thus protecting wounds from infections and ensuring unrestricted transportation of gas and liquid molecules. We have described several polymers in this study that have been used to create scaffolds made of electrospun nanofibers. These scaffolds are studied and discussed using different polymers to show the effect on skin repair mechanisms and investigate the remodeling abilities aiming to potentially show a foundation for clinical applications and industrial manufacturing. The extracellular matrix (ECM) and the nanofiber structure share many similarities, and the use of different types of polymers, including biopolymers like collagen and chitosan and biodegradable polymers like polycaprolactone, polylactic acid, and polyvinyl alcohol, helps to make the field relevant to skin regeneration and remodeling. Hence, this review summarized and discussed the polymeric nanofibers such as collagen, polycaprolactone, poly vinyl alcohol reporting pre-clinical trials of wound healing and skin regeneration.

Keywords: wound healing, nanofibers, skin remodeling, polymers, multifunctional scaffolds, skin regeneration

1. Introduction

The skin is considered the largest organ in the human body that is functionalized to protect the human systems against mechanical, chemical, and thermal stress, microbial/pathogenic invasion, and prevent dehydration. Accordingly, the large surface area of the skin can be associated with several conditions such as cutaneous wounds of acute or pathological conditions which represent significant challenges clinically and socioeconomically. It has been statistically proven in the year 2003 that globally over 6 million patients suffer from severe skin burns each year and among which more than 300,000 patients lose their fight against burn pain and pass away ultimately [1–4]. It has globally shown an economic burden of over 9.5 billion US dollars a year [5, 6]. Wound healing delay or impairment is considered a global health issue with affects people suffering from comorbid diseases such as diabetes, cardiovascular diseases, cancer, and obesity. Non-healing wounds have shown negative impacts on patients' life that includes different aspects from the quality of life, pain, and well-being psychological distress to physical discomfort [5, 7, 8]. As reported in 2014, 6.0% of the United Kingdom and 9.3% of the United States populations were diagnosed with diabetes which will indicate a global rise of diabetic adults to 439 million by 2030 [5, 6, 9]. This is related to the hospitalizations of diabetic foot ulcers, infection complications, amputations, and mortality of patients [6, 9]. Thus as a result of wounds with diabetes and obesity, the incidence of pressure and venous ulcerations is expected to rise in the upcoming years as a consequence of the aging of the population that is estimated to increase up to 60% in Europe population will be aged above 65 by 2050 and obesity that will exceed 20% of obese world's adults by 2030 [5, 6, 9, 10]. Hemostasis, inflammation, proliferation, and remodeling are the four distinct but overlapping stages of the multistage biological process of wound healing. A proper biomaterial must be created to support the intricate skin architecture. The synthetic biomaterial scaffold must resemble the ECM and be resilient to the biological, topographical, and physicochemical characteristics of natural skin tissue [11]. As a result, traditional therapies for wound management have been urged for the need for advanced and more effective strategies to control the wound status, preventing invasive solutions to save the patients [8]. The era of biomaterial technology that has been rapidly developing recently has shown huge potential for clinical application including skin remodeling, tissue engineering, and wound healing. A large number of excellent biomaterials either naturally or synthetically have shown various advantages over traditional therapies [4, 8, 12, 13]. Mainly biomaterials include PLA, PCL, PVA, PEG, PEO, collagen, hyaluronic acid, sodium alginate, chitosan, gelatin, etc. [1–4, 7, 8, 10, 13–15,]. Electrospinning and nanofibers formation have been the subject of intensive studies and research in multiple fields among is tissue-engineering. This is correlated to the large surface area to volume ratio and the high porosity of the nanofibers formed web [4, 8, 14–16,]. Thus, the biomedical application of nanofibers in wound care contributes not only to the physical protection of wound sites from infection and pathogenic sources due to the properties of high surface area and porosity of nanofibers but also provides an excellent environment for soft tissue regeneration and skin remodeling due to the nature of several biodegradable polymers which modulate the gaseous exchange of the wound location and help in promoting hemostasis while also preventing the scar formation of the skin [4, 8, 10, 12–14, 16].

In this study, we have reported several materials that have been used to produce electrospun nanofibers scaffolds. These scaffolds are studied and discussed using different polymer-nanofibers scaffolds to show the effect on skin repair mechanisms and investigate the remodeling abilities aiming to potentially show a foundation for clinical applications and industrial manufacturing.

2. Tissue scaffold and drug delivery

The unique properties of nanofibers from high surface area and wide porosity helped in the application of nanofibers in mechanical engineering and biological tissue scaffolds. Thus, the selection of the tissue scaffolding material is carefully selected to guarantee the biocompatibility of the human cells with it. The material properties have shown great influence on the biocompatibility of the surface chemistry of the scaffolds [13, 17, 18]. The mechanical support of the skin is regulated by several things rising from biological signals of growth factors, ECM, and the surrounding cells [17–19]. The responsible cells and growth factors vary from primary and secondary elements of ECM, among which are collagen, and natural polymers of different types: Types I and III which are considered primary structural elements of ECM that functionalized in supporting the tissue reconstruction [19]. The high surface area to volume ratio that nanofibers excel in, helps in the cell attachment which provides a regenerative tissue scaffold [17–21]. The natural ECM and its dimensional have been adapted to perform the scaffold of bioengineered polymers in the same manner. The variability of biodegradable polymers such as PLGA, PCL, etc.... are commonly used in electrospinning tissue engineering as they tend to produce highly structured tissue scaffolds with high porosity of both pore diameter and pore volume [4, 11, 17–20, 22].

The electrospun nanofiber scaffolds that tend to have high porosity ease the passage of nutrient intake and metabolic exchange as the space provided for the cell to accommodate these activities is enough. For the use of electrospun nanofibers as tissue scaffolds, mechanical characteristics such as the modulus of elasticity and strain at failure are crucial. By altering the solution concentration and fiber orientation, the material characteristics may be appropriately tailored [4, 11, 13, 20, 21, 23]. In a study carried out by Matthews and his team where they investigated the usage of Collagen Type I from calfskin and Types I and III from the human placenta to produce electrospun nanofibers. Results have shown that the electrospun collagen fibrils were tightly resembling the natural polymer tissue properties of both structural and biological. These electrospun collagen microfibrils allowed the cultivation of aortic muscle cells, which resulted in scaffolds with a high density of smooth muscle cells. The investigation has proven that the electrospun collagen revealed the presence of highly interwoven muscle cells [17, 21]. In another study, Huang and his team constructed an experiment on electrospun nanofibers of collagen and PEO mats to show their potentiality in wound healing and tissue engineering. The result was the production of uniform fibers with diameters between 100 and 150 nm. The significant intermolecular contact between the PEO and collagen component was assumed due to the better mechanical characteristics of the collagen nanofibers [17, 23].

Nanofiber mats are used as drug carriers in drug delivery systems, due to their great functional qualities. With biocompatible delivery matrices made of either biodegradable or nonbiodegradable polymers, controlled drug delivery at a set rate throughout a predetermined treatment time is conceivable [17, 22]. In a study carried out by Kenawy and his team investigating the potential of electrospun polymers PEVA, PLA with ethanol, and tetracycline hydrochloride as a drug delivery system. The results have shown that the release of tetracycline from electrospun fibers was much greater than from the casted films. The observations of electrospun PEVA AND 50/50 PLA/PEVA fibers have shown a very consistent release of tetracycline over the investigated period of 5 days [17, 22]. The previously stated studies have shown the necessity of applying nanofibers mats in controlled DDS and biomedical sectors. When administered to the skin, these medications with nanofiber as demonstrated in **Figure 1**, the incorporation can promote wound healing or just simple drug release for systemic or local therapeutic activity.

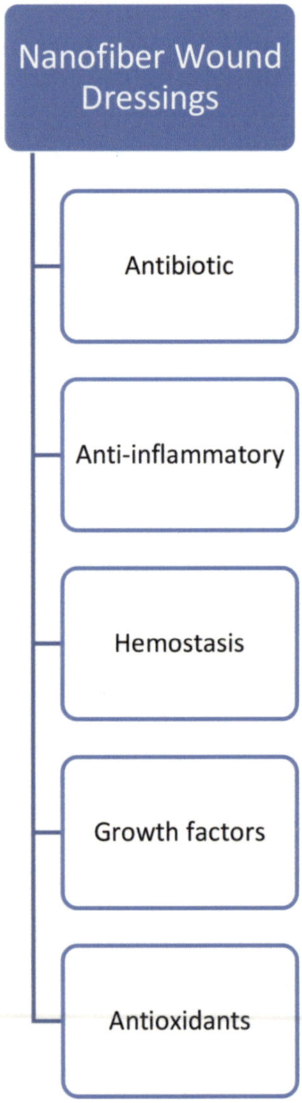

Figure 1.
Schematic illustrating various types of pharmaceutical agents that can be incorporated into nanofibers for wound dressings.

2.1 Nanofibers scaffolding for wound healing

Scaffolds may be easily modified in situ during the electrospinning process or thereafter to be suited for a particular biomedical application with the usage of electrospinning [13, 24]. The choice of polymer, which determines the mat's rate of degradation, can be used to influence the rate at which a drug or drugs are released from a nanofiber mat or the positioning of the drug within or on the surface of the fibers [4, 13, 22, 24, 25]. Information on choosing a polymer is supplied, along with several strategies for customizing the active agent's position inside the electrospun mat [11, 13, 24]. Rapid hemostasis and effective antibacterial properties are the two key criteria for acceptable present-day wound dressings. The goal of a wound dressing is to quickly achieve hemostasis, and it should also have powerful antibacterial properties in order to protect against bacterial infections from the surroundings. Due of its flexibility in creating nanofibrous membranes for wound dressing that can provide a moist environment surrounding the wound region that promotes healing, electrospinning has gained an enormous amount of interest [4, 13, 24, 26].

2.1.1 Selection of polymers to enhance wound healing mechanisms

The suitable polymer matrix, whether natural, synthetic, or a combined mix of polymers, should be used when developing nanofiber mats for wound healing applications in order to meet the necessary scaffold qualities. Utilizing nanofiber-based systems, several natural and synthetic chemicals have recently been tested for their ability to improve and enhance the healing of wounds [24, 27]. Among the most investigated electrospun nanofibers is an organic based polymer, PCL because it supports faster healing and decreases inflammatory infiltration, PCL, a biodegradable and biocompatible poly(a-ester), has been extensively studied and used for tissue regeneration and wound healing applications. PCL is a useful matrix for loading natural compounds like curcumin, herbal extracts, and proteins because of its significant physico-chemical features, including hydrophobic qualities, great spinnability, favorable mechanical properties, and delayed degradation [10, 14, 28]. Several studies have investigated PCL nanofibers alone and drug loaded. Thus, in a study conducted in 2015 by Ana Delia Pinzon-Garcia and her team investigating Bixin-loaded PCL nanofibers, as PCL has tendency of incorporating the insoluble medications and may be employed in a variety of formulations for controlled drug administration and tissue engineering. The study noticed that animals treated with Bix-PCL1 nanofiber and Bix-PCL2 nanofiber showed a much higher percentage of wound closure. According to their finding, even while Bixin release from PCL nanofibers promoted wound healing from the first days on and was more effective than PCL alone, increasing Bixin concentration on PCL's more hydrophobic nanofibers created an unfavorable environment for wound healing. Here, they showed that the most effective concentration of Bixin in the nanofibers to induce an efficient rapid wound closure was 2.5% [24, 28]. In another study, Sang-Myung Jung and his team investigated the natural extract of Spirulina loaded with electrospun PCL nanofibers on animal model. The in vivo testing showed how the nanofiber affected skin, which reacted intricately with different substances. The team applied the Spirulina extract PCL nanofibers directly to the full thickness wound and assessed its effects, which showed a fast reduction in the size of the lesion. In particular, the average size of the groups varied starting on day 5 and persisted until day 10. These outcomes proved that spirulina extract-PCL nanofibers had the same effects in vivo as it did in vitro [29]. In a further studied PCL-loaded nanofiber Robin and his Indian team, investigated the capacity of ZnO nanoparticles to produce ROS, which may have a function in biological systems, is well established. Through growth factor-mediated pathways, ROS can promote cell adhesion and migration to speed up wound healing. Hence, the study has discussed the creation of ZnO nanoparticle-infused electrospun PCL scaffolds and their potential to serve as materials that can replace skin and speed up the healing process. In guinea pigs, subcutaneously implanted PCL membranes with or without ZnO nanoparticles were tested. Studies in immunology, macroscopy, and histology have demonstrated that using membranes containing ZnO nanoparticles improves cell adhesion and migration. The membranes with implanted ZnO nanoparticles do not exhibit any adverse reactions of irritation. The implant also improved wound healing without the development of scars [30].

Other highly studies polymer is PLA, that is selected in various studies as the supporting material because it is biodegradable, biocompatible, and can support the proliferation and attachment of various cells promoting the healing process of the skin. It is possible to employ the patterned PLA surfaces as a platform for the targeted transport and engraftment of different type of cells such as stem cells [31–34]. In a study investigated the usage of PLA with other nanofibrous scaffolds by Marziyeh Ranjbar-Mohammadi's team, the design of electrospun composite nanofibers using natural nano-fibrillated chitosan /ZnO nanoparticles combination as the nanofiller ingredient has been examined during this study. The key components are PLA and K/PVA. K/PVA/Chitosan ZnO (2:1)-PLA/Chitosan ZnO (2:1) nanofiber, with a diameter of 352.50 ± 31 nm, a contact angle of 48 ± 3°, and a tensile strength of 0.96, 0.18 MPa, is proposed as a suitable wound healing scaffold with the greatest antibacterial and ability to enhance cell proliferation [31]. Additionally, as PLA nanofibers are biocompatible and have a large specific surface area and high porosity, they were employed in the study carried out by Thuy Thi Thu Nguyen's team to study the PLA as a carrier for Cur to improve its functional characteristics. Cur/PLA blended nanofibers with various concentrations of Cur were studied for their chemical and biological properties. Cell adhesion and proliferation are promoted by the inclusion of Cur in the blended nanofibers, even at concentrations as low as 0.125 weight percent. A mouse model was used to test the in vivo wound healing capabilities of Cur-loaded PLA nanofibers. When compared to PLA nanofibers (58%), treatment with Cur-loaded PLA nanofibers dramatically enhanced the rate of wound closure (87%) on day 7. The findings of this study indicate that Cur-loaded nanofibers have shown no adverse actions and increased the potential of using PLA loaded curcumin in wound healing patches [32]. In another study conducted in Italy by Giulia Milanesi, electrospun PLA and essential oil nanofibers were then covered with medium-molecular-weight chitosan to enhance the antibacterial effect of EO. Before electrospinning, BP-EO or L, both of which are known for having antibacterial properties, were added to the PLA/acetone solution. The results showed that the CS coating improved the fibrous mats' hydrophilicity, increased EO's antibacterial potential, and encouraged cell adhesion and proliferation [35]. Also, in a study carried out in 2015 in Prague, Czech Republic on AA-collagen poly lactic acid nanofiber scaffold investigating how human dermal fibroblast adhesion and proliferation were affected by fibrin placed on a nanofibrous membrane and AA added to the cell culture medium. The study findings demonstrated that compared to the membrane lacking fibrin, fibrin deposition led to noticeably better cell adherence and spreading. While the cells on the membranes with fibrin were polygonal in form and widely dispersed with well-developed characteristic FA carrying 1-integrins, the cells on the membranes without fibrin were spherical until the third day of cell culture. The adherence of fibroblasts to fibrin molecules is mediated by 1-integrins, namely 51 integrins (together with v3 and v3 integrins), in which these adhesion receptors recognize the RGD motifs. The collagen receptors 11, 21, and 31 integrins are also members of the group of integrins to fibrin-coated membranes, particularly in the medium with AA, collagen expression and synthesis increased, which may have contributed to the enhanced cell adhesion to the modified PLA membranes. Additionally, the fibrin pulls molecules of ECM from the cell culture media through its C domain, including fibronectin and vitronectin, which help to enhance cell attachment even more. Cell adhesion on unaltered membranes is essentially solely mediated by spontaneously adsorbed ECM molecules from the cell culture medium or by cell deposition on the membrane surface. Additionally, these compounds could be adsorbed insufficiently and with the incorrect spatial configuration for cell adhesion receptor recognition. The research demonstrated that AA boosted collagen I expression and induced cells to deposit collagen fibers on material surfaces. The cells grown in a typical cell culture media (without AA) did not significantly develop collagen ECM on the surface of the material. Collagen I was expressed more strongly by the cells grown in the regular culturing medium on membranes coated with fibrin than by the cells grown in the medium with AA on membranes without coating. On the material surface, however, these cells did not significantly deposit a fibrous collagen matrix. The study had proven that human dermal fibroblasts were significantly impacted by the fibrin nanocoating on PLA nanofibrous membranes. Fibrin boosted the expression of 1-integrins, cell proliferation, and collagen production while promoting cell adhesion and spreading. Fibrin likely had a positive impact on cell adhesion and proliferation because of its simplicity in binding to cells via integrin adhesion receptors, which attracted sticky molecules from the cell culture media. It was possibly also because of the cells' mitogenic properties. Collagen I's mRNA expression, the total amount of collagen produced, and its deposition as ECM on the membrane surface were all boosted by fibrin [11, 36].

Further, the well-known PVA is a synthetic polymer that is water soluble, non-toxic, biocompatible, and biodegradable. PVA has so received much research in the domains of biomedicine, polymers, and textiles. PVA resins offer a wide range of practical uses due to their outstanding chemical resistance, physical characteristics, and biocompatibility, including fibers for clothing and industry, adhesives and binders, films, membranes, materials for drug delivery systems, and embolic materials that destroy cancer cells. Due to the use of water-based solvents, PVA electrospinning has been the subject of much research. PVA was therefore selected as an appropriate foundation polymer to create an electrospun nanofibrous structure [37–42]. In a study conducted in 2020 in Iran investigating the PVA nanofibers anti-bacterial efficacy when loaded with anti-biotic drug, the study's primary objective was to create wound dressings utilizing the electrospinning technique and a mixture of TXA and PVA to examine the blood coagulation capabilities. Additionally, CTX and PVA were blended to take into account their antibacterial capabilities. The findings of a study on the antibacterial activities of Gram-negative (*Escherichia coli*) and Gram-positive (*Staphylococcus aureus*) bacteria showed that the antibacterial characteristics grew stronger with rising MIC. 100% was achieved in PVA/CTX dressing with MIC: 8 g/ml. PVA-TXA dressings (10 mg/ml) and (20 mg/ml) both showed adequate blood coagulation abilities. PVA-TXA (20 mg/ml) exhibited a stronger blood coagulation ability with an average absorption of 0.031. The results have proven the ability of PVA nanofibers to enhance the wound healing mechanism specially when loaded with certain concentrations of TXA and CTX [37]. Herein, in another study by Sama Ghalei and her team, a new nanocomposite wound dressing was created implementing electrospun PVA nanofibers and nanoparticles that can release the medication DLF at the wound site. They said that because the structure combines the beneficial qualities of both polymeric nanofibers and NPs, it is extremely promising. Due to the drug-loaded NPs' insoluble nature in the original PVA solution, the hydrophilic PVA nanofibers may also be used to load and release the hydrophobic DLF. The electrospun composite dressing made of zein nanoparticles and PVA nanofibers has a tremendous potential for use in the treatment of wounds, according to the results [43]. Also, in a study conducted in early 2012, electrospinning was used to create CS aqueous salt combined with PVA nanofiber mats. Without using harmful or toxic solvents, CS was dissolved in distilled water along with HOBt, TPP, and EDTA. In an in vivo wound healing test, the CS-HOBt/PVA and CS-EDTA/PVA nanofiber mats showed satisfactory antibacterial activity against both gram-positive and gram-negative bacteria, and the CS-EDTA/PVA nanofiber mats outperformed gauze in reducing acute wound size in the first week following tissue damage. The study has suggested the significance of the CS-EDTA/PVA nanofiber mats to be used as wound dressing materials since they are biodegradable, biocompatible, and antibacterial [44].

Moving forward to natural based polymers, starting with one of the most prevalent natural polysaccharides is chitosan, a partly N-deacetylated derivative of chitin. Chitosan is the only naturally occurring alkaline polysaccharide with positive charge that has been identified so far. It is made up of random mixes of -(1-4)-linked d-glucosamine and N-acetyl-d-glucosamine in the polymer backbone. Due to its excellent biocompatibility, biodegradability, antibacterial, and anti-inflammatory properties, chitosan-based biomaterials have attracted considerable attention recently. After cellulose, chitosan is the most prevalent biopolymer on earth. Shrimp and other crustacean shells are used to extract chitosan. There have been reports of other extraction techniques, however the deacetylation of chitin is the most often used. As a biopolymer, chitosan has several functions and applications. However, altering its chemical structures can improve its mechanical, chemical, and biological properties [45–48]. In a study carried out in 2009 on chitosan combined with silver nanoparticles. The study investigated the electrospinning CS/PEO solutions containing Ag/CS colloids with in-situ chemical reduction of Ag ions, fairly homogeneous CS/PEO ultrafine fibers containing silver nanoparticles were effectively created. The research demonstrated the efficacy of CS/PEO and Ag/CS/PEO nanofibers with a 1:1 mass ratio of CS/PEO against *E. coli*. The antibacterial activity of the nanofibers containing Ag nanoparticles was superior to that of the CS/PEO nanofibers. For Ag/CS/PEO nanofibers containing 1.1 and 2.2 wt% nanoparticles, respectively, all bacteria were inactivated within 10 and 6 hours. Ag/CS/PEO membranes have shown extremely potent antibacterial properties that might be employed in a variety of biomedical applications, including tissue scaffolds, body wall repairs, wound dressings, and antimicrobial filters [49]. Additionally, in an interesting study that as conducted on natural extracts in order to create a biocompatible, antibacterial nanofibrous wound dressing, two natural extracts were loaded onto synthetic honey, PVA, and chitosan nanofibers. The HPCS nanofibers in the HPCS-CE, HPCS-AE, and HPCS-AE/CE nanofiber mats, respectively, were loaded with dried aqueous extract of Cleome droserifolia (CE) and dried aqueous extract of *Allium sativum* (AE). By demonstrating improved wound closure rates in mice and by histologically examining the wounds, a preliminary in vivo result found that the produced nanofiber mats improved the wound healing process when compared to the untreated control. Additionally, the HPCS and HPCS-AE/CE showed similar effects on the wound healing process when compared to the commercial dressing the study referred to, however the HPCS/AE allowed for a faster rate of wound closure. Results of studies on cell cultures demonstrated that the created nanofiber mats were more biocompatible than the commercial product the study referred to, which displayed pronounced cytotoxicity. The study significantly proven that the natural nanofiber mats that have been produced have an opportunity to be effective, biocompatible, antibacterial wound dressings [50]. Consequently, the other natural polymer that is extensively studied in the wound-care management is collagen, an attractive polymer for the creation of wound dressings since it is a biopolymer and a significant component of ECM. These include minimal immunogenicity, strong biocompatibility, hemostatic qualities, the capacity to stimulate cellular proliferation and adhesion, non-toxicity, and low antigenicity. The ECM of various sensitive tissues is mostly made up of collagen. All dermal dry materials, which are located at the skin's level in proportions of 70–80 percent, define the presence of collagen. Collagen promotes the maintenance and differentiation of cellular phenotypes, hence interactions between collagen and cells are crucial for the process of wound healing. Collagen-based nanofibers have also showed intriguing features that are useful in the fields of skin regeneration and wound dressings [51–53]. In a research study conducted by Cheng-Hung Lee 's team investigating the capabilities of Collagen nanofibers in diabetic wounds. The team produced nanofibrous collagen/PLGA scaffold membranes, which allowed for the sustained release of Glucophage for diabetic wounds. The development of glucophage-loaded collagen/PLGA nanofibrous membranes that sustainably provided medication to treat diabetic wounds. For more than 3 weeks, the team has proven that the nanofibrous membranes emitted significant amounts of glucophage. In their finding, they have stated that the collagen/PLGA membranes coated with glucophage significantly accelerated the healing of diabetic lesions. Additionally, due to the downregulation of matrix metalloproteinase 9, the collagen content of diabetic rats employing drug-eluting membranes was greater than that of the control rats. According to the experimental findings presented by the team, glucophage-loaded collagen/PLGA membranes with a nanofibrous structure were proved successful in promoting early wound healing in diabetic wounds and increasing collagen content [51, 54].

3. Conclusion

Due to its ease of use and ability to be combined with other techniques, electrospinning, while being a rather old process, has maintained its significance. Electrospinning, which is the most reliable size for native ECM, allows material characteristics to be controlled down to the nanoscale level. The approach to building nanofiber scaffolds from a single polymer, many mixed polymers, or various inputs may be adapted with the help of changes in the electrospinning equipment and process parameters. Due to the development of novel polymers and manufacturing techniques, multifunctional wound dressing scaffold materials with adaptable surface functions and exceptional structural and mechanical characteristics are now feasible. Bio-based polymeric materials have frequently been advocated for skin tissue regeneration in a variety of wound healing settings as useable skin substitutes, useful dressings, and wound healing patches. As many functional biomaterials, superabsorbent dressings, multifunctional wound dressings, and skin tissue scaffold materials are launched in place of traditional gauzes, the need for bioinspired wound care solutions is growing. Potential wound care solutions will need to offer a variety of unique biological capabilities, such as biomimetic, bio-responsive, antibacterial, and hemostatic qualities, to establish a favorable microenvironment. The anticipated efficacy in wound healing scaffolds will be closer to reality as more current biopolymers are studied for their physicochemical, biological, and mechanical characteristics, as well as when new ones are created. Studies employing nanofibers for tissue engineering purposes have multiplied exponentially to date. This paper mainly discussed the most recent advancements employing different skin-remodeling polymers for wound healing and skin regeneration. Numerous research has shown that natural bio-macromolecules are legitimate substitutes for their synthetic equivalents when it comes to wound treatment, as was covered in this review. More intriguingly, the ability to electrospun fibers into nanostructures by applying nano-structuring enables the development of biomimetic dressings with enhanced bioactivity for stimulating tissue regeneration. Different wound models have been used in in vitro and in vivo testing to demonstrate the effectiveness of electrospun dressings made of natural/synthetic polymeric materials in promoting cell migration and proliferation, speeding wound closure, regulating the inflammatory response, and, in certain circumstances, avoiding the formation of biofilms. However, difficulties in electrospinning some materials are related to the following: choosing the proper solvents or polymer additives to facilitate fiber extrusion; the requirement of postprocessing procedures to improve the mechanical resistance and control the scaffolds' rate of degradation. Importantly, in terms of fiber shape and dimensionality, the scaffold's design is biomimetic for the natural ECM, and its likely functions as an immediate short-term matrix for hemostatic activities and skin remodeling cells that assist wound healing. Electrospun nanofiber scaffolds have shown to be very adaptable. The interactions that took place at the interface between the materials' surface and biology may be controlled by adjusting the matrix chemistry, surface functionality, and mat degradation rate in combination. Natural, semi-synthetic, and completely synthetic polymer-based nanofibers and their composites have demonstrated promise as materials for skin regeneration and scaffolding for wound healing. Nanofiber scaffolds have a position in wound care therapy because they resemble natural ECM shape and structure both on their own and when combined with other functional polymers. This provides a good environment (niche) for skin tissue rebuilding. Systematic investigations are also required to standardize fabrication techniques under hygienic electrospun settings to gradually transition nanofibers from the laboratory to the commercial scale. As previously discussed throughout the review, tissue regeneration and skin remodeling are subjective to the degree of stress/wound and the causes of such injuries which result in the selection of a certain polymer whether natural or synthetic source that can itself act as ECM or can be loaded with various substances such as antibiotics, hemostatic agents, growth factors, antioxidants, and anti-inflammatory. As a result, the nanofiber mat may be employed as an effective skin substitute material that will accelerate cell migration and proliferation to heal wounds quickly. The review suggests carrying out more clinical investigations while considering the patient acceptability of the administration form to improve the incorporation of appealing medications into nanofibers and using a combination of various biopolymers. The challenge of scaling up to mass manufactures of polymeric or drug-loaded electrospun mats must also be taken into account.

Notes/thanks/other declarations

Thanks to my beloved parents Hatem ElGamal and Lilian Ibrahim for their continual love and support.

Acknowledgements

This work is supported by the research and development department of Eva Pharma. The author acknowledges support from the director of the department Laila Gad ElRub and the manager of the transdermal and patches sector Bassem Samy Shenouda. The author is grateful for their guidance, ongoing discussions, critical suggestions, and knowledge in the era of biomaterials. My apologies to all the investigators, researchers, and scientists in the area whose publications were not cited in this overview. This can only be a small sample of the many excellent works that are accessible in the literature.

Conflict of interest

The author declares no potential conflicts of interest with respect to the research and/or publication of this work.

Acronyms and abbreviations

ECM	Extracellular matrix
PLA	Polylactic acid
PCL	Poly caprolactone
PVA	Poly vinyl alcohol
PEG	Poly ethylene glycol
PEO	Poly ethylene oxide
PLGA	Poly lactic-glycolic acid
PEVA	Poly ethylene co-vinyl acetate
DDS	Drug Delivery System
Bix-PCL	Bixin-loaded PCL
ZnO	Zinc Oxide
ROS	Reactive oxygen species
K	Keratin
nm	Nanometer
MPa	Mega Pascal
Cur	Curcumin
EO	Essential oil
AA	Ascorbic acid
CS	Chitosan
BP-EO	Black pepper-essential oil
L	Limonene
TXA	Tranexamic acid
CTX	Ceftriaxone
DLF	Diclofenac
NPs	Nanoparticles
HOBt	Hydroxybenzotriazole
TPP	Thiamine pyrophosphate
EDTA	Ethylenediaminetetraacetic acid
Ag	Silver
HPCS	Synthetic-honey chitosan nanofibers
CE	Cleome droserifolia
AE	*Allium sativum* aqueous extract

Author details

Farida ElGamal
Evapharma Research and Development, Cairo, Egypt

*Address all correspondence to: faridahatem1424@gmail.com

References

[1] Madison KC. Barrier function of the skin: "la raison d'etre" of the epidermis. Journal of Investigative Dermatology. 2003;**121**(2):231-241

[2] Brandner JM, Jensen JM. The skin: An indispensable barrier. Experimental Dermatology. 2008;**17**:1063-1072

[3] Jin G, Prabhakaran MP, Kai D, Annamalai SK, Arunachalam KD, Ramakrishna S. Tissue engineered plant extracts as nanofibrous wound dressing. Biomaterials. 2013;**34**(3):724-734

[4] Akombaetwa N, Bwanga A, Makoni PA, Witika BA. Applications of electrospun drug-eluting nanofibers in wound healing: Current and future perspectives. Polymers. 2022;**14**(14):2931

[5] Gould LJ, Fulton AT. Wound healing in older adults. Rhode Island Medical Journal. 2016;**99**(2):34

[6] Jung K, Covington S, Sen CK, Januszyk M, Kirsner RS, Gurtner GC, et al. Rapid identification of slow healing wounds. Wound Repair and Regeneration. 2016;**24**(1):181-188

[7] Yan X, Yu M, Ramakrishna S, Russell SJ, Long YZ. Advances in portable electrospinning devices for in situ delivery of personalized wound care. Nanoscale. 2019;**11**(41):19166-19178

[8] Mele E. Electrospinning of natural polymers for advanced wound care: Towards responsive and adaptive dressings. Journal of Materials Chemistry B. 2016;**4**(28):4801-4812

[9] Hruby A, Hu FB. The epidemiology of obesity: A big picture. PharmacoEconomics. 2015;**33**:673-689

[10] Green DW, Ben-Nissan B, Yoon KS, Milthorpe B, Jung HS. Bioinspired materials for regenerative medicine: Going beyond the human archetypes. Journal of Materials Chemistry B. 2016;**4**(14):2396-2406

[11] Behere I, Ingavle G. In vitro and in vivo advancement of multifunctional electrospun nanofiber scaffolds in wound healing applications: Innovative nanofiber designs, stem cell approaches, and future perspectives. Journal of Biomedical Materials Research Part A. 2022;**110**(2):443-461

[12] Chen H, Zhang H, Shen Y, Dai X, Wang X, Deng K, et al. Instant in-situ tissue repair by biodegradable PLA/ Gelatin nanofibrous membrane using a 3D printed handheld electrospinning device. Frontiers in Bioengineering and Biotechnology. 2021;**9**:684105

[13] Ji Y, Song W, Xu L, Yu DG, Annie Bligh SW. A review on electrospun poly (amino acid) nanofibers and their applications of hemostasis and wound healing. Biomolecules. 2022;**12**(6):794

[14] Chong EJ, Phan TT, Lim IJ, Zhang YZ, Bay BH, Ramakrishna S, et al. Evaluation of electrospun PCL/gelatin nanofibrous scaffold for wound healing and layered dermal reconstitution. Acta Biomaterialia. 2007;**3**(3):321-330

[15] Ghosal K, Agatemor C, Tucker N, et al. Electrical spinning to electrospinning: A brief history. In: Electrospinning: basic research to commercialization. Royal Society of Chemistry. 2018

[16] Pereira RF, Barrias CC, Granja PL, Bartolo PJ. Advanced biofabrication strategies for skin regeneration and repair. Nanomedicine. 2013;**8**(4):603-621

[17] Subbiah T, Bhat GS, Tock RW, Parameswaran S, Ramkumar SS. Electrospinning of nanofibers. Journal of Applied Polymer Science. 2005;**96**(2):557-569

[18] Li WJ, Laurencin CT, Caterson EJ, Tuan RS, Ko FK. Electrospun nanofibrous structure: A novel scaffold for tissue engineering. Journal of Biomedical Materials Research: An Official Journal of The Society for Biomaterials, The Japanese Society for Biomaterials, and The Australian Society for Biomaterials and the Korean Society for Biomaterials. 2002;**60**(4):613-621

[19] Young DS. Hyaluronic acid-based nanofibers via electrospinning.

[20] Boland ED, Wnek GE, Simpson DG, Pawlowski KJ, Bowlin GL. Tailoring tissue engineering scaffolds using electrostatic processing techniques: A study of poly (glycolic acid) electrospinning. Journal of Macromolecular Science, Part A. 2001;**38**(12):1231-1243

[21] Matthews JA, Wnek GE, Simpson DG, Bowlin GL. Electrospinning of collagen nanofibers. Biomacromolecules. 2002;**3**(2):232-238

[22] Kenawy ER, Bowlin GL, Mansfield K, Layman J, Simpson DG, Sanders EH, et al. Release of tetracycline hydrochloride from electrospun poly (ethylene-co-vinylacetate), poly (lactic acid), and a blend. Journal of Controlled Release. 2002;**81**(1-2):57-64

[23] Huang L, Apkarian RP, Chaikof EL. High-resolution analysis of engineered type I collagen nanofibers by electron microscopy. Scanning. 2001;**23**(6):372-375

[24] Rieger KA, Birch NP, Schiffman JD. Designing electrospun nanofiber mats to promote wound healing–a review. Journal of Materials Chemistry B. 2013;**1**(36):4531-4541

[25] Su Y, Su Q, Liu W, Jin G, Mo X, Ramakrishn S. Dual-drug encapsulation and release from core–shell nanofibers. Journal of Biomaterials Science, Polymer Edition. 2012;**23**(7):861-871

[26] Liu M, Duan XP, Li YM, Yang DP, Long YZ. Electrospun nanofibers for wound healing. Materials Science and Engineering: C. 2017;**76**:1413-1423

[27] Kamble P, Sadarani B, Majumdar A, Bhullar S. Nanofiber based drug delivery systems for skin: A promising therapeutic approach. Journal of Drug Delivery Science and Technology. 2017;**41**:124-133

[28] Pinzón-García AD, Cassini-Vieira P, Ribeiro CC, de Matos Jensen CE, Barcelos LS, Cortes ME, et al. Efficient cutaneous wound healing using bixin-loaded PCL nanofibers in diabetic mice. Journal of Biomedical Materials Research Part B: Applied Biomaterials. 2017;**105**(7):1938-1949

[29] Jung SM, Min SK, Lee HC, Kwon YS, Jung MH, Shin HS. Spirulina-PCL nanofiber wound dressing to improve cutaneous wound healing by enhancing antioxidative mechanism. Journal of Nanomaterials. 2016;**1**:2016

[30] Augustine R, Dominic EA, Reju I, Kaimal B, Kalarikkal N, Thomas S. Electrospun polycaprolactone membranes incorporated with ZnO nanoparticles as skin substitutes with enhanced fibroblast proliferation and wound healing. RSC Advances. 2014;**4**(47):24777-24785

[31] Ranjbar-Mohammadi M, Shakoori P, Arab-Bafrani Z. Design and characterization of keratin/PVA-PLA nanofibers containing hybrids of nanofibrillated chitosan/

ZnO nanoparticles. International Journal of Biological Macromolecules. 2021;**187**:554-565

[32] Nguyen TT, Ghosh C, Hwang SG, Tran LD, Park JS. Characteristics of curcumin-loaded poly (lactic acid) nanofibers for wound healing. Journal of Materials Science. 2013;**48**:7125-7133

[33] Foldberg S, Petersen M, Fojan P, Gurevich L, Fink T, Pennisi CP, et al. Patterned poly (lactic acid) films support growth and spontaneous multilineage gene expression of adipose-derived stem cells. Colloids and Surfaces B: Biointerfaces. 2012;**93**:92-99

[34] Evans GR, Brandt K, Katz S, Chauvin P, Otto L, Bogle M, et al. Bioactive poly (L-lactic acid) conduits seeded with Schwann cells for peripheral nerve regeneration. Biomaterials. 2002;**23**(3):841-848

[35] Milanesi G, Vigani B, Rossi S, Sandri G, Mele E. Chitosan-coated poly (lactic acid) nanofibres loaded with essential oils for wound healing. Polymers. 2021;**13**(16):2582

[36] Bacakova M, Musilkova J, Riedel T, Stranska D, Brynda E, Zaloudkova M, et al. The potential applications of fibrin-coated electrospun polylactide nanofibers in skin tissue engineering. International Journal of Nanomedicine. 2016;**11**:771

[37] Fatahian R, Mirjalili M, Khajavi R, Rahimi MK, Nasirizadeh N. Fabrication of antibacterial and hemostatic electrospun PVA nanofibers for wound healing. SN Applied Sciences. 2020;**2**:1-7

[38] Yao L, Haas TW, Guiseppi-Elie A, Bowlin GL, Simpson DG, Wnek GE. Electrospinning and stabilization of fully hydrolyzed poly (vinyl alcohol) fibers. Chemistry of Materials. 2003;**15**(9):1860-1864

[39] Lee JS, Choi KH, Ghim HD, Kim SS, Chun DH, Kim HY, et al. Role of molecular weight of atactic poly (vinyl alcohol) (PVA) in the structure and properties of PVA nanofabric prepared by electrospinning. Journal of Applied Polymer Science. 2004;**93**(4):1638-1646

[40] Koski A, Yim K, Shivkumar SJ. Effect of molecular weight on fibrous PVA produced by electrospinning. Materials Letters. 2004;**58**(3-4):493-497

[41] Zhang C, Yuan X, Wu L, Han Y, Sheng J. Study on morphology of electrospun poly (vinyl alcohol) mats. European Polymer Journal. 2005;**41**(3):423-432

[42] Son WK, Youk JH, Lee TS, Park WH. Effect of pH on electrospinning of poly (vinyl alcohol). Materials Letters. 2005;**59**(12):1571-1575

[43] Ghalei S, Asadi H, Ghalei B. Zein nanoparticle-embedded electrospun PVA nanofibers as wound dressing for topical delivery of anti-inflammatory diclofenac. Journal of Applied Polymer Science. 2018;**135**(33):46643

[44] Charernsriwilaiwat N, Rojanarata T, Ngawhirunpat T, Opanasopit P. Electrospun chitosan/polyvinyl alcohol nanofibre mats for wound healing. International Wound Journal. 2014;**11**(2):215-222

[45] Cui C, Sun S, Wu S, Chen S, Ma J, Zhou F. Electrospun chitosan nanofibers for wound healing application. Engineered Regeneration. 2021;**2**:82-90

[46] Negm NA, Hefni HH, Abd-Elaal AA, Badr EA, Abou Kana MT. Advancement on modification of chitosan biopolymer and its potential applications. International Journal of Biological Macromolecules. 2020;**152**:681-702

[47] Rodríguez-Rodríguez R, Espinosa-AndrewsH,Velasquillo-MartínezC, García-Carvajal ZY. Composite hydrogels

based on gelatin, chitosan and polyvinyl alcohol to biomedical applications: A review. International Journal of Polymeric Materials and Polymeric Biomaterials. 2020;**69**(1):1-20

[48] Ding F, Deng H, Du Y, Shi X, Wang Q. Emerging chitin and chitosan nanofibrous materials for biomedical applications. Nanoscale. 2014;**6**(16):9477-9493

[49] An J, Zhang H, Zhang J, Zhao Y, Yuan X. Preparation and antibacterial activity of electrospun chitosan/poly (ethylene oxide) membranes containing silver nanoparticles. Colloid and Polymer Science. 2009;**287**:1425-1434

[50] Sarhan WA, Azzazy HM, El-Sherbiny IM. Honey/chitosan nanofiber wound dressing enriched with Allium sativum and Cleome droserifolia: Enhanced antimicrobial and wound healing activity. ACS Applied Materials & Interfaces. 2016;**8**(10):6379-6390

[51] Lee CH, Singla A, Lee Y. Biomedical applications of collagen. International Journal of Pharmaceutics. 2001;**221**(1-2):1-22

[52] Mbese Z, Alven S, Aderibigbe BA. Collagen-based nanofibers for skin regeneration and wound dressing applications. Polymers. 2021;**13**(24):4368

[53] Zhang L, Webster TJ. Nanotechnology and nanomaterials: Promises for improved tissue regeneration. Nano Today. 2009;**4**(1):66-80

[54] Lee CH, Chang SH, Chen WJ, Hung KC, Lin YH, Liu SJ, et al. Augmentation of diabetic wound healing and enhancement of collagen content using nanofibrous glucophage-loaded collagen/PLGA scaffold membranes. Journal of Colloid and Interface Science. 2015;**439**:88-97

Chapter 7

Fabrication Techniques for Scaffolds Applied in Regenerative Medicine

Mekha Grace Varghese, Annie Thomas, Rupesh S, Sameer KM, Derick Joseph, Aby Mathew T and Nebu George Thomas

Abstract

Tissue engineering strategies in regenerative medicine combine cells, scaffolds, and growth factors to regenerate and reconstruct pathologically damaged tissues such as periodontium, bone, nerves, cartilage skin, heart valves, and various other organs. Scaffolds have a major role as they provide a three-dimensional environment for tissue regeneration. They act as an extracellular matrix that favors the ingrowth of new cells thereby assisting the regeneration of target tissues. Various properties of scaffolds like scaffold architecture, surface topography, biodegradability, mechanical properties, and manufacturing process are important to achieve optimal results in tissue engineering. Scaffold fabrication can be achieved by conventional as well as non-conventional current manufacturing techniques. Solvent casting, phase separation, particulate-leaching, gas foaming, freeze-drying, and electrospinning are conventional methods for fabricating scaffolds. The architecture of these scaffolds greatly depends on processing techniques. Fused deposition modeling, hydrogel processing, selective laser sintering, decellularization techniques, three dimensional printing, and bioprinting, are current techniques for scaffold fabrication. The chapter will give an overview of each fabrication technique and will aid biomedical engineers to select the ideal fabrication technique for specific applications in the field of regenerative medicine.

Keywords: electrospinning, fused deposition modeling, rapid prototyping, scaffold fabrication, stereolithography, three-dimensional bioprinting, tissue engineering

1. Introduction

Regenerative medicine is a broad field that focuses on self-healing and tissue engineering is an integral part of it. Langer and Vacanti have described tissue engineering as "an interdisciplinary field that applies the principles of engineering and life sciences toward the development of biological substitutes that restore, maintain, or improve function or a whole organ" [1]. Generally, three strategies are adopted for the creation of new tissues: cells or cell substitutes, tissue-inducing substances, and cells placed on or within matrices known as scaffolds [2]. Scaffolds are engineered to cause desirable cellular interactions thereby contributing to the formation of new

Premade porous scaffolds	Decellularised extracellular matrix	Cell sheets	Cell encapsulated in hydrogel
Raw materials fabricated into porous scaffolds	Decellularised native tissues	ECM secretion on confluent cells forms cell sheets	Cell mixing on monomer solution
↓	↓	↓	↓
Cells seeded to form cell seeded scaffolds	Porous scaffolds	Laminated to multiple cell sheets	Cell encapsulated in hydrogel
↓	↓	↓	↓
Implantation	Cell seeded scaffolds	Implantation	Injection
	↓		
	Implantation		

Table 1.
Different scaffolding approaches in tissue engineering.

functional tissues. They mimic the extra-cellular matrix and form a microenvironment that serves purposes like cell attachment, migration, diffusion of vital nutrients, etc. The clinical success of tissue engineering largely depends upon scaffold architecture, material composition, and fabrication techniques.

The specific requirements that a scaffold must-have is as follows. They should have high porosity and appropriate pore size to enable active cell seeding and nutrient diffusion. They should be biodegradable with a degradation rate similar to the tissue formation rate. Adequate structural integrity is needed to maintain a three-dimensional environment. Both synthetic and natural materials are used for scaffold fabrication. The synthetic ones include polylactic acid (PLA) [3], polyglycolic acid (PGA), polycaprolactone (PCL), and poly-lactic-co-glycolic acid [4] each with its tailored degradation rates. The tunability and biocompatibility are advantageous for scaffold fabrication [4]. Natural materials can be proteinaceous such as collagen and fibrin or polysaccharides like chitosan and glycosaminoglycans (GAG). Decellularised tissues may also function as scaffolds. They are formed by chemically extracting cells from tissues leaving behind an extracellular matrix but can possess serious immunologic complications (**Table 1**).

2. Scaffold fabrication

The design and fabrication of scaffolds depend upon the mechanical, biological, and physicochemical requirements of the scaffold. The pore size, pore interconnectivity, degradation statistics, stability, etc. are taken into consideration during the fabrication process [5]. The 2D scaffold fabrication is more accurate and easy with good control over the physicochemical properties. Fabrication of 3D scaffolds is challenging and requires advanced bio-printing and bio assembly which is automated. Computer assisted designing and machining technologies help in such 3D designs as sponges, meshes, and foams. 3D technologies have further revolutionized into 4D printing techniques which are quite expensive.

Several scaffold fabrication techniques have been described so far based on the biomaterial used, the tissue intended to regenerate as well as the purpose of the scaffold. The techniques can be broadly classified into conventional and advanced types.

3. Conventional techniques

Conventional fabrication technologies include solvent casting/ particle leaching, thermally induced phase separation, gas forming, freeze drying, melt molding, sol-gel method and electrospinning [6].

3.1 Solvent casting/particle leaching

Here, a polymer is dissolved in a highly volatile solvent into which a porogen is uniformly distributed. The porogen can be an organic compound like gelatin, collagen, or glucose microspheres or inorganic water soluble salts like KCl or NaCl. The polymer-solvent-porogen mixture is cast into a mold. When the solvent is evaporated, a composite network of polymer with entrapped porogen is obtained. Then using a suitable solvent, the porogen is dissolved which creates a porous scaffold. The porosity can be altered by altering the composition of the polymer mixture or the volume fraction of porogen.

The technique produces scaffolds with a degree of porosity between 50–90% and pore sizes ranging from 5 to 600 μm. The pore sizes can also be tuned by altering the porogen content or its size and shape [7]. The process is relatively easy and of low cost. The long processing time, variations in pore interconnectivity, and poor mechanical properties are the disadvantages [8]. The thickness of the scaffold is also limited. Hazards from residual solvent may also be anticipated.

3.2 Thermally induced phase separation/TIPS

The polymer to be used like PLA is dissolved in an easily sublimable solvent with a low melting point like dioxane. The mixture is then quenched to induce phase separation and polymer rich and polymer poor phases are formed. When the mixture is cooled below the melting point of the solvent and then subjected to vacuum drying, sublimation takes place leaving behind a porous scaffold. The scaffolds obtained have high porosity of more than 90% with uniform pore size and good pore interconnectivity. But uniform pore distribution cannot be attained and the reproducibility of scaffolds is also unattainable [6]. Since the technique uses lower temperatures and there is the complete removal of the organic solvent, TIPS is particularly employed for bioactive heat labile drugs. Thermoplastics are mainly processed by the TIPS technique. The process is relatively inexpensive also.

3.3 Gas foaming

This technique uses pressurized and non-pressurized gases instead of organic solvents for porosity formation. In the polymer solution, gases are introduced by in situ generation of gas bubbles known as nucleation. Nucleation can be achieved by a chemical blowing agent or by a physical blowing agent. Agents like sodium bicarbonate act as chemical blowing agents whereas gases like nitrogen and carbon dioxide are used as physical blowing agents [9]. The evolution of gases results in void formation and formation of a porous matrix.

By this method, hazards related to the organic solvents are eliminated. Highly porous scaffolds are obtained with the preservation of the bioactive species. Porosity is approximately 85% and pore size is approximately 100μm. This method applies to both hydrophobic and hydrophilic polymers [10]. The disadvantages include lack of precise control over pore size and poor pore interconnectivity. The processing time is also longer [11].

3.4 Freeze drying/Lyophilisation

In freeze drying, a polymer solution is prepared by dissolving the polymer in an organic solvent or organic solvent-water emulsion. The polymer solution is mold cast and frozen below its triple point by liquid nitrogen or by refrigeration. The frozen mixture is then subjected to two step drying process. The primary and secondary drying by sublimation removes the formed ice crystals and pores are formed in their places [12].

It's a commonly used method where almost dry and highly porous scaffolds with high interconnectivity are made. The porosity obtained is more than 90% and pore sizes range from 20 to 200 μm. Irregular pore sizes are obtained but pore sizes can be controlled by altering the temperature, drying time or polymer concentration. The procedure is expensive and time consuming [13].

3.5 Melt molding

This is the technique used for thermoplastic polymers where the polymers are melted and cast into a suitable 3D mold. The structure of the mold conforms to the defect. Porosity will be introduced by methods like gas foaming or particulate leaching. Later, the scaffolds are freeze dried. Most commonly used polymer for melt molding is PLGA due to its low glass transition temperature. PLGA is mixed with gelatin microspheres and cast in a Teflon mold. The mold is then heated above the glass transition temperature of PLGA which allows the incorporation of biomaterial through the gelatin forming a composite. The composite is then placed in water so that the water soluble microspheres get dissolved leaving behind a porous structure [14].

The method is simple with precise control over pore size and pore interconnectivity. There is no use of organic solvents that is detrimental to cell growth and differentiation. The disadvantage is that thermolabile drugs cannot be incorporated because of the high temperatures during melt molding [15].

The most commonly used strategy in melt molding is the injection molding technique. It's a highly economical, productive and flexible technique.

3.6 Sol-gel method

The principle behind the sol-gel process is hydrolysis and polycondensation. The precursors are organic or inorganic metal compounds like metal alkoxides or metal chlorides. These are dissolved in water or organic solvent where they undergo hydrolysis and polycondensation to form a colloid solution. The resultant solution is then cast into 3D molds. The low viscosity of sol makes it easier to cast into any particular shape. Then in the 3D mold, the gelation process starts with interactions between the contents forming 3D networks. The resultant product is dried in the mold itself and later subjected to gentle heating for solidification of the matrix. Dehydration or chemical stabilization is done later to create ultra-stable porous material [16].

This technique uses low temperatures but longer processing time and the high cost of the raw materials precludes its wide application. The sol-gel method is particularly employed for the fabrication of bioactive glasses and bioceramics.

3.7 Electrospinning

The most commonly employed technique to produce nanofibers is electrospinning. In this spinning, technique electrostatic forces are used to produce fibrous scaffolds from biocompatible polymers. It's a rapid and simple technique where high voltage electric current is applied to a molten polymer solution that is extruded out of a fine needle. The ultra-fine polymer fibers thus generated are deposited on a grounded collector. The method uses two electrodes, one placed into the spinning polymer solution and the other attached to the collector. When an electric charge is applied to the molten polymer contained in the capillary tube, a charged jet of fluid is ejected. The discharged jet solidifies when traveling in the air and forms a polymer fiber that is deposited onto a grounded metallic collector [17].

The formed scaffold mimics the extracellular matrix and has a high surface to volume ratio. Electrospinning can process a wide range of polymers and can fabricate micro and nano scaffolds with high porosities.

4. Advanced techniques/rapid prototyping (RP)

Rapid prototyping comprises those advanced manufacturing processes that enable the creation of tailor-made patient-specific scaffolds useful in tissue engineering. This unique process helps in the direct manufacturing of scaffolds from data obtained by computer aided designing (CAD) models, CT or MRI. RP is also known as solid free-form fabrication or additive manufacturing. Since there is a layer-by-layer deposition of the material, precise spatial control is possible over the polymer structure and desirable mechanical properties can be achieved [18].

The first 3D printing technology was reported by Hull et al, in 1986. They described a 3D scaffold fabrication technique that used UV light exposure for layer-by-layer fabrication of constructs [19]. Because it's a layer-by-layer fabrication technique, the precision of constructs was high, unlike the conventional procedure. Over the years, other additive manufacturing techniques were developed.

The basic technique is as follows. A computer aided three-dimensional design of the scaffold is produced preferably from the data obtained through CT or MRI. The design is then transferred to a standard tessellation language (STL) [14] format where it can be sliced into thin horizontal cross-sections. The resultant data obtained is then transferred to the RP machine which fabricates the scaffold by layer-by-layer deposition of the polymer material.

4.1 Stereolithography

Stereolithography is an additive manufacturing technique that solidifies resin into 3D scaffolds by photopolymerization. The principle of stereolithography is the selective curing of a photosensitive resin/polymer by using an ultraviolet [20] laser. The main components of the system are a tank containing photosensitive liquid polymer, a built platform for depositing the cured resin, a UV laser for radiation and a dynamic mirror system. With the help of UV laser, a layer of photosensitive resin is deposited on the platform. Once the initial layer is deposited and solidified, the platform is lowered vertically and a second layer is placed over the first layer. In this manner, a 3D scaffold is created. After cleaning off the uncured resin, post curing is done for the scaffold using UV light. The process uses data from an STL file, where a 3D model is converted into 2D slices, based on which layer-by-layer deposition occurs.

The curing reaction of resin is an exothermic reaction that is initiated by UV light. During the curing process, two transition stages are noticed – gelation and vitrification. In gelation, the liquid resin changes to rubbery consistency with increased viscosity. In vitrification, the rubber resin changes to glassy solid resin [21].

Four generations of stereolithography approaches have been described so far. The first generation technique described by Hull uses a laser beam to cure the liquid resin [19] the second generation technique is known as projection stereolithography where each layer is simultaneously cured by photo mask technology. Here, once a thin layer of resin is deposited, the resin is illuminated through a photo mask for curing. The uncured portions are removed, refilled with resin and again cured. The process is repeated until the desired pattern is obtained. The need for several masks and the precision required during mask alignment makes this a time consuming process and therefore less desirable [22].

In 2015, Tumbleton et al, described the third generation approach which is the continuous lithography technique. It is based on continuous liquid interface production (CLIP) with which the print speed of scaffolds can be reduced from hours to minutes [23]. A recent innovation in this context is the volumetric stereolithography that fabricates 3D geometries and is useful in processing high viscous resins.

Uniformity in pore structure and pore interconnectivity can be obtained. The viability of cells and the presence of growth factors can be maintained. The technique is quite expensive.

4.2 Selective laser sintering (SLS)

An additive manufacturing technique in which laser is used as the heat source to fuse the powder particles is known as SLS. This is also a layer-by-layer formation technique based on computer assisted pre-designed architectures. A computer controlled laser beam like a CO_2 laser is used on powdered materials. The heat from the laser sinters/ fuses the powder and this continues in a layer-by-layer manner to build 3D constructs. Cells or biomaterials cannot be incorporated into scaffolds due to the higher temperature involved [9].

High precision and control over scaffold fabrication are possible with a high degree of porosity and mechanical strength. Only thermally stable materials can be processed by this method. Removal of residual material is also tedious as the compound materials are in powdered form [24].

4.3 Fused deposition modeling (FDM)

The most popular and widely used additive manufacturing technique is fused deposition modeling. They are used for metals and thermoplastic materials. Here, a temperature controlled extruder and nozzle help in depositing the thermoplastic material onto a platform to produce 3D scaffolds. The material in the form of filament is driven through the extruder using rollers and gets converted into a molten form. Through the nozzle, a thin layer is deposited precisely and sequentially. The extrusion and deposition are entirely under the control of a computer aided tool. The deposition takes place on the surface of a base that is movable vertically which allows it to be lowered after the deposition of each layer, thereby adding more layers on top. Layer-by-layer deposition of the thin filament takes place which cools on exposure to air resulting in the fusion of these filaments to form scaffolds of desired 3D architecture [9].

The scaffolds obtained have high mechanical strength and a high degree of porosity. The size and structure of the pores can be adjusted [25]. As the technique uses high temperatures, non-thermoplastic materials cannot be processed by FDM.

4.4 Three dimensional bioprinting

A recently developing technology that uses bioinks and living cells to print 3D structures is bioprinting. In this additive manufacturing technique also, layer-by-layer development of tissues and organs is accomplished in a bottom-up manner. Every attempt is made to mimic the normal tissues in both form and function. Advantages include the creation of patient-specific tailor-made constructs which mimic the concerned tissues or organs. Since the process is automated, precision can be achieved in the organization of cells and extracellular matrix. Layer-by-layer construction also ensures good pore interconnectivity. But the technique is also expensive and complex [26]. The bio ink used for bioprinting is a composite made of cells and other biomaterials. They can also be made from natural and synthetic polymers such as alginate, collagen, hydroxyapatite, polyethylene glycol,l etc.

The different strategies involved in 3D bioprinting are ink-jet printing, extrusion printing, and laser assisted bioprinting [27]. The basic steps in all strategies are the same with a pre-processing, processing and post-processing phases. In the pre-processing stage, the bio images of the target tissue are obtained via CT or MRI, followed by the construction of accurate 3D models using CAD. The data thus obtained will be converted to 2D stacks based on which the bio ink is selected and fed to the bioprinter. In the processing phase, actual bioprinting is done in a layer-by-layer manner using any of the four strategies mentioned earlier. Post-processing phase is a maturation phase in a bioreactor, followed by structural and functional characterization of the constructs [28].

Bioprinting can be done as a scaffold based and scaffold free approach. In the scaffold based approach, the cellular deposition takes place on a biomaterial matrix in the form of a 3D construct. The construct should closely mimic the extracellular matrix so that cells will grow and populate it. In scaffold free approach, cells or tissues will be directly laid down to form patterns like spheroids or honeycombs [29].

4.4.1 Ink-jet based bioprinting

In this type, the bioink is deposited over a biopaper substrate. The technique is digitally controlled and has a non-contact printing pattern. Two ways of ink-jet printing are continuous ink-jet printing and the drop-on-demand (DOD) technique [30].

In continuous ink-jet (CIJ) printing, pressure is applied on the bioink to force it out of a nozzle as a continuous jet. The ejected jet is subjected to an electric field to deflect it onto a substrate. The excess droplets are deflected to a gutter for collection and re-use. In DOD inkjet printing, the droplets are produced on demand. Instead of the continuous pressure CIJ method, here a pulsed pressure is used. DOD technique is more favored because there is no reuse of the bioink as in the CIJ method, thereby avoiding the risk of contamination [31].

The DOD technique is further categorized into two types, thermal method and piezoelectric method. In thermal method, a pulsed electric current is applied to a heating element that vaporizes the ink creating pressure by the vapor. This pressure forces the bioink through the nozzle onto the substrate [32]. But in the piezoelectric method, a pulsed voltage is applied onto the piezoelectric transducer that creates pressure. Exposure to high temperatures is occurring only for a few microseconds and so the viability of cells is not compromised [33]. The printing characteristics depend on the viscosity of the ink and the size of the droplets, which in turn depends on factors like nozzle size, nozzle to substrate distance, temperature gradient, frequency of current etc.

4.4.2 Extrusion based bioprinting

This is a direct ink writing method where the material is continuously extruded out of the nozzle for layer-by-layer deposition and the creation of 3D architecture. Here, either mechanical force from a piston or pneumatic forces are used for extrusion of bioink through the nozzle onto the substrate. The whole process is computer controlled and produces small streams of bioink in contrast to the droplets of inkjet method [34]. This technique is favorable for highly viscous bioink types and also for high cell densities. The drawback is that the high forces for extrusion may affect cell viability and distorts the cellular structures [20].

4.4.3 Laser assisted 3D bioprinting

This is a non-contact direct writing method where the deposition of bioink onto the substrate is facilitated by a pulsed laser beam. The three main elements of laser assisted technique are a pulsed laser source, a ribbon coated with heat sensitive bioink and a substrate for printing [30]. Laser source can be UV or near UV wavelength lasers. Volatilization of the bioink on the ribbon takes place with the application of laser which propels a high speed jet of cell laden bioink onto the substrate. The substrate here is a plate made of quartz or materials that allows laser transmission [35].

Sometimes, a sacrificial interlayer is placed between the bioink and the ribbon, which has laser absorbing properties, thereby assisting in maintaining cell viability. Coating the substrate surface with a natural biopolymer can also help, by facilitating cell attachment and growth. The two approaches described are the LIFT and MAPLE DW. LIFT uses high energy pulsed laser whereas the latter uses a low powered pulsed laser. In LIFT, the sacrificial layer is made of metal or metal oxides. High energy pulsed laser can cause rapid thermal expansion of this sacrificial layer that causes high speed propulsion of bioink onto the substrate. Biological laser processing or BioLP is a variant technique where the sacrificial layer is a hydrogel.

The living cells can either be embedded inside the polymeric matrix or imprinted onto the matrix. The viability of cells is affected by the energy of the laser, the thickness of sacrificial layer and the viscosity of bioink. Thicker sacrificial layers and viscous bioink favored cell viability whereas higher energy of laser compromised it.

The factors to be considered during 3D bioprinting are the following. The choice of bioink should be accurate to favor the formation of a desirable 3D structure. Low viscosity bioinks should be preferred as high viscosity bioinks can compromise the cell viability during the extrusion process [36]. Most of the systems can only print one type of bioink during one deposition process. Attempts including the use of multi nozzle bioprinters were tried to extrude different types of bioink during a single deposition process. Moreover, the structure once printed cannot transform itself in response to biological stimuli. This is in contrast to the nature of native tissues that are highly responsive and dynamic [37]. Taking all these into consideration happened the emergence of four dimensional printing techniques.

5. Four dimensional printing

Four dimensional printing is the most advanced technology for the fabrication of multi material scaffolds. They are tailor-made and patient-specific with the potential to change shape over time [38]. They are mostly made of those materials that respond to stimuli and undergo dynamic configuration in response. Thus, they are of high use in large bony defects. Their development is still in infancy, because of challenges like the need to cope with the dynamic transformation of native tissues [38].

6. Conclusion

Since tissue engineering is an interdisciplinary field, the developments happening in scaffold fabrication techniques have an important role in determining success in this field. The fabrication techniques have evolved from conventional ones to the current 3D bioprinting methods where tissues and organs are engineered. Each technique has its pros and cons. 3D printing technology has and will play an important role in the field of scaffold development. But the development of a scaffold that can match the dynamic responses of the native tissues is still unattained. Studies related to the nanoarchitecture of the scaffolds as well as the incorporation of bioactive molecules and their sustained release are still in their infancy and are areas of potential research.

Conflict of interest

The author declares no conflict of interest.

Author details

Mekha Grace Varghese[1*], Annie Thomas[2], Rupesh S[3], Sameer KM[4], Derick Joseph[5], Aby Mathew T[6] and Nebu George Thomas[7]

1 Pushpagiri Research Center, Pushpagiri Institute of Medical Sciences, Thiruvalla, Kerala, India

2 Department of Prosthodontics, Annoor Dental College, Muvattupuzha, Kerala, India

3 Department of Pediatric and Preventive Dentistry, Malabar Dental College and Research Centre, Edappal, Kerala, India

4 Department of Periodontics, M.E.S Dental College, Perinthalmanna, Kerala, India

5 Department of Conservative Dentistry and Endodontics, PSM Dental College, Thrissur, Kerala, India

6 Department of Prosthodontics, Pushpagiri College of Dental Sciences, Thiruvalla, Kerala, India

7 Department of Periodontics, Pushpagiri College of Dental Sciences, Thiruvalla, Kerala, India

*Address all correspondence to: mekhagrace@gmail.com

References

[1] Langer R, Vacanti J. Tissue engineering. Science. 1993;**260**(5110):920-926. DOI: 10.1126/science.8493529

[2] Turnbull GC, Picard J, Riches F, Jia P, Han L, Li F, et al. 3D bioactive composite scaffolds for bone tissue engineering. Bioactive Materials. 2017;**3**:278-314. DOI: 10.1016/j.bioactmat.2017.10.001

[3] Chan BP, Leong KW. Scaffolding in tissue engineering: General approaches and tissue-specific considerations. European Spine Journal. 2008;**17**(Suppl. 4):467-479

[4] Gentile P, Carmagnola I, Hatton PV. An overview of poly(lactic-co-glycolic) acid (PLGA)-based biomaterials for bone tissue engineering. International Journal of Molecular Sciences. 2014;**15**(3):3640-3659. DOI: 10.3390/ijms15033640. PMC 3975359

[5] Bhushan S et al. Scaffold fabrication techniques of biomaterials for bone tissue engineering: A critical review. Bioengineering. 2022;**9**(12):728

[6] Zhao P, Mi H, Rao C, Fu J, Turng LS. Fabrication of scaffolds in tissue engineering: A review. Frontier in Mechanical Engineering. 2018;**13**:107-119

[7] Li Z, Li Y, Ma Y, Li J-S, Dai F-Y. Recent progress in tissue engineering and regenerative medicine. Journal of Biomaterials and Tissue Engineering. 2016;**6**(10):755-766

[8] Adel IM, ElMeligy MF, Elkasabgy NA. Conventional and recent trends of scaffolds fabrication: A superior mode for tissue engineering. Pharmaceutics. 2022;**14**:306

[9] Devi GVY, Anil S, Venkatesan J. Biomaterials and scaffold fabrication techniques for tissue engineering applications. In: Sheikh FA, editor. Engineering Materials for Stem Cell Regeneration. Singapore: Springer Singapore; 2021. pp. 691-706

[10] Salerno A et al. Design of porous polymeric scaffolds by gas foaming of heterogeneous blends. Journal of Materials Science. Materials in Medicine. 2009;**20**(10):2043-2051

[11] Reddy MSB et al. A comparative review of natural and synthetic biopolymer composite scaffolds. Polymers (Basel). 2021;**13**(7):1105

[12] Morais AR et al. Freeze-drying of emulsified systems: A review. International Journal of Pharmaceutics. 2016;**503**(1-2):102-114

[13] Collins MN et al. Scaffold fabrication technologies and structure/function properties in bone tissue engineering. Advanced Functional Materials. 2021;**31**(21):2010609

[14] Mabrouk M, Beherei HH, Das DB. Recent progress in the fabrication techniques of 3D scaffolds for tissue engineering. Materials Science & Engineering. C, Materials for Biological Applications. 2020;**110**:110716

[15] Allaf R. Melt molding technologies for 3D scaffold in Functional 3D Tissue Engineering Scaffolds: Materials, T., and Applications. Cambridge, UK: Woodhead Publishing; 2017. pp. 75-100

[16] Preethi Soundarya S et al. Bone tissue engineering: Scaffold preparation using chitosan and other biomaterials with different design and fabrication techniques. International Journal of Biological Macromolecules. 2018;**119**:1228-1239

[17] Smith JA, Mele E. Electrospinning and additive manufacturing: Adding three-dimensionality to electrospun scaffolds for tissue engineering. Frontiers in Bioengineering and Biotechnology. 2021;**9**:674738

[18] Abdalla Eltom GZ, Muhammad A. Scaffold techniques and designs in tissue engineering functions and purposes: A review. Advances in Materials Science and Engineering. 2019;**2019**, Article ID 3429527:13. DOI: 10.1155/2019/3429527

[19] National Center for Biotechnology Information. PubChem Patent Summary for US-6027324-A, Apparatus for production of three dimensional objects by stereolithography. 2024. Retrieved 4 February 2024. Available from: https://pubchem.ncbi.nlm.nih.gov/patent/US-6027324-A

[20] Guvendiren M et al. Designing biomaterials for 3D printing. ACS Biomaterials Science & Engineering. 2016;**2**(10):1679-1693

[21] Da Silva bartolo PJ, editor. Stereolithography: Materials, Processes and Applications. London: Springer Nature; 2011

[22] Huang J, Wang J. A review of stereolithography: Processes and systems. PRO. 2020;**8**(9):1138. DOI: 10.3390/pr8091138

[23] Tumbleston JR et al. Continuous liquid interface production of 3D objects. Science. 2015;**347**(6228):1349-1352

[24] Du Y, Yang Q, Wang S, Wang J, Ma J, et al. Selective laser sintering scaffold with hierarchical architecture and gradient composition for osteochondral repair in rabbits. Biomaterials. 2017;**137**:37-48

[25] Dhinakaran V, Ram PB, Ravichandran M, Vinayagamoorthy M. A review on recent advancements in fused deposition modeling. Materials Today Proceedings. 2020;**27**:752-756

[26] Agarwal S et al. Current developments in 3D bioprinting for tissue and organ regeneration: A review. Frontiers in Mechanical Engineering. 2020;**6**:589171

[27] Murphy S, Atala A. 3D bioprinting of tissues and organs. Nature Biotechnology. 2014;**32**:773-785. DOI: 10.1038/nbt.2958

[28] Papaioannou TG, Manolesou D, Dimakakos E, Tsoucalas G, Vavuranakis M, Tousoulis D. 3D bioprinting methods and techniques: Applications on artificial blood vessel fabrication. Acta Cardiology Sinica. 2019;**35**(3):284-289. DOI: 10.6515/ACS.201905_35(3).20181115A

[29] Ozbolat IT. Bioprinting scale-up tissue and organ constructs for transplantation. Trends in Biotechnology. 2015;**33**(7):395-400

[30] Bishop ES et al. 3-D bioprinting technologies in tissue engineering and regenerative medicine: Current and future trends. Genes & Diseases. 2017;**4**(4):185-195

[31] Alamán J et al. Inkjet printing of functional materials for optical and photonic applications. Materials. 2016;**9**(11):910

[32] Dababneh AB, Ozbolat IT. Bioprinting technology: A current state-of-the-art review. Journal of Manufacturing Science and Engineering. 2014;**136**(6):061016

[33] Cui X, Boland T, D'Lima D, Lotz K. Thermal inkjet printing in tissue engineering and regenerative medicine. Recent Patents on Drug Delivery & Formulation. 2012;**6**(2):149-155

[34] Panwar A, Tan LP. Current status of bioinks for micro-extrusion-based 3D bioprinting. Molecules. 2016;**21**(6):685

[35] Guillotin B et al. Laser assisted bioprinting of engineered tissue with high cell density and microscale organization. Biomaterials. 2010;**31**(28):7250-7256

[36] Jakus AE, Rutz AL, Shah RN. Advancing the field of 3D biomaterial printing. Biomedical Materials. 2016;**11**(1):014102

[37] Burdick JA, Murphy WL. Moving from static to dynamic complexity in hydrogel design. Nature Communications. 2012;**3**:1269

[38] Li YC et al. 4D bioprinting: The next-generation technology for biofabrication enabled by stimuli-responsive materials. Biofabrication. 2016;**9**(1):012001

Chapter 8

Application of Hydroxyapatite in Regenerative Dentistry

Prameetha George Ittycheria, Thomas George, Mathew John, G. Meenu, Vimal Thomas, S. Aswathy, Rene Kuriakose and Jerin Thomas

Abstract

In clinical practice, dentists face alveolar bone loss that needs to be managed by bone grafts. The basic bone grafting materials are autograft, allograft, xenograft, and alloplasts. Autografts are gold standard because it has osteoconduction osteoinduction osteogenic. However, they possess risk for the morbidity of the donor site and limited availability. Allograft have possibility of disease transmission and immunologic reactions. These problems potentiated the use of alloplasts. For bone regeneration, hydroxyapatite is the reference material because of its biocompatibility, bioactivity, osteoconductivity, and osteoinductive property. Natural hydroxyapatite can be synthesized from fishbone, coral, bovine bone, eggshell, and seashells. Hydroxyapatite bone substitute has ideal properties for socket preservation, sinus augmentation, periodontal regeneration and in restorative and preventive dentistry. When used as implant coatings, they support osseointegration and osteogenesis. Hydroxyapatite known for its bone regenerative capacity. Nano-hydroxyapatite, with smaller size and wider surface area, permits more proteins and cells to attach to the surface speed up regeneration. Hydroxyapatite are used as inorganic building blocks for tissue engineering or as nano-fillers with polymers. Furthermore, ion doping and surface modifications have been reported to prepare functionalized hydroxyapatite. This chapter illustrates the role of hydroxyapatite in regenerative dentistry, and advances and advantages of using it as a component of other dental materials, whether experimental or commercially available.

Keywords: natural hydroxyapatite, bone regeneration, restorative dentistry, scaffold, dental materials

1. Introduction

Hydroxyapatite (HAp)—the key inorganic element of teeth and bones [1, 2]. It is extensively used in dental clinics and for bone repair, because its good biocompatibility and biological activity. Nanohydroxyapatite (nHA) a type of nanomaterial having small crystal grain diameter, wider surface interface, high surface and binding energy. Nano-hydroxyapatite act as a drug carrier to deliver anti-tumor drugs [3]. High hardness and wear-resistance of tooth enamel depends on the braidedinorganic-organic composite structure and multilayer structure [4]. The natural remineralizing ability of hydroxyapatite is still restricted, but numerous studies have shown a high promoting effect on remineralization. There mineralizing performance is further improved by the introduction of acidic amino acids and flouride. To speed up the drug absorption and to treat periodontal diseases such as jaw cyst, HAp paste is effectively used [5]. Nano-hydroxyapatite with porous microspheres have numerous benefits such as high drug load,large specific surface area, better biocompatibility, pH-responsive degradation, used in tumor detection and tumor drug carrier, in bone repair, the combination of HA with natural and synthetic polymers has effectively solved problems such as high brittleness and uncontrollable degradation rate" [5].

2. Shortcomings of available bone regenerative materials

A bone graft material's main purpose is to aid osseous healing by providing a cellular environment for new bone creation, a structural framework during the healing process. Tissue viability, defect size, graft size, shape, and volume, biomechanical features, graft handling, cost, ethical considerations, biological traits, and associated repercussions all factor into the optimum bone graft selection [6]. Bone graft material has different attributes for regeneration and they vary according to the graft material used (**Table 1**) [7].

The materials utilized in grafting of bone can be classified into different categories mainly autografts, xenografts, and allografts. Other types include biologically and synthetic based biomaterials, tissue-engineered biomaterials, and combination of these substitutes (**Table 2**).

The grafts mentioned above has its own set of benefits and drawbacks. Following are the shortcomings of available bone regenerative materials (**Table 3**).

After decades of research works on the best available regenerative materials, studies have reached a prime focus on naturally available resources. Out of which naturally available hydroxyapatite has gained much attention compared to readily available synthetic grafts due to its predictable results. Hydroxyapatite is a natural polymer of calcium phosphate derived from bone or natural materials such as coral, algae, fishes and other marine sources and commonly utilized to accelerate

Attribute	Description
Osteogenic	Ability to differentiate and produce bone
Osteoinductive	Provide a biologic stimulation (proteins and growth factors) that causes mesenchymal stem cells and other osteoprogenitor cells to proceed into the osteoblast lineage
Osteoconductive	Allow for cellular attachment, proliferation, and migration by providing a structure and topography that allows for cell attachment, proliferation, and migration
Osteointegrative [8]	Forms tenacious bond formed between the new mineralized tissue & graft material

Table 1.
Attributes of bone grafts [7].

Type	Description
Autografts	Because of osteogenic, osteoconductive, and osteoinductive capabilities, along with the lack of foreign body responses, they are the bench mark. Obtained from intra oral and extra oral sites.
Allografts	Biological materials obtained from the same species. Primarily serve as an osteoconductive or structural matrix, but they lack osteoinductive qualities.
Xenografts	Bone substitutes derived from other species like bovine or swine grafts, and transplanted into humans having osteoconductive property
Alloplasts	Synthetic bone graft substitutes having osteoconductive property

Table 2.
Various kinds of bone grafts [9–11].

Bone graft	Short comings
Autograft [9–14]	Needs second surgery so surgical morbidity and discomfort, possibility of surgical complications, ankylosis and root resorption, limited graft volume
	Cortical bone grafts-higher resorption rate, less vasculature, resulting in less bone remodeling
	Cancellous bone grafts-mechanically weak
Allografts [11–14]	Infection and allograft fracture due to decreased revascularization, possibility of transmission of disease, sterilization of graft may compromise its osteoinductive potential, high cost of procurement, the host's immune reaction, inconsistency of graft integration, high failure rate, expensive, due to ethical and legal concerns.
Xenograft [11–17]	Antigenicity, tissues must be handled carefully to eliminate organic components, unpredictability of regeneration and resorption rates
Alloplasts [11–17]	Demineralized bone matrix-lack of structural stiffness caused by processing and the difficulty to locate the material radiographically due to its intrinsic lucency. Ceramics are not osteoinductive, compressive strengths are lower than cortical bone

Table 3.
Shortcomings of bone regenerative materials.

bone repair owing to its potential to operate as a structural scaffold. Because chemical composition of hydroxyapatite closely mirrors that of bone's inorganic component, it can be employed as a superior biocompatible bone grafting material. Natural HA is less expensive, and the key raw ingredient is readily available. Natural HA shows substitutions and traces of certain chemical elements due to which its bioactivity behavior can be enhanced, compared with that of synthetic HA. Also this kind of substitutions promotes the formation of noval bone. Natural HA is considered as a better regenerative material than synthetic Hap due to its bone bonding ability, significant biocompatibility mediated by its porous architecture [11–18].

Although synthetic HA is widely known for its capacity to link with bone tissue, it is restricted due to its reduced solubility, sluggish rate of bone binding ability, and bacterium adhesion inhibition. This is a significant disadvantage since patient recuperation is hampered, and infection can result in surgical failure. Because HA's crystal structure is porous, it can easily accommodate ion replacements. Due of its increased crystallinity and Ca/P ratio, synthetic HA has a very low resorption rate.

Another important issue with HA is its low mechanical strength, which prevents it from being employed in high-load-bearing applications [11–17].

3. Clinical application of hydroxyapatite in alveolar bone regeneration

Many grafting materials are used in dentistry which include allograft, autograft, alloplastic and xenograft graft. The advantages and short comings are mentioned above in this chapter.

Since then there is an interest in the use of alloplastic (synthetic) grafting materials.

The first synthetic bone graft that was used in 1892 by Van Meekeren, who treated bone defect as using calcium sulfate. Since then, materials classified under bioceramics are substituted as bone grafts in humans. The conventional bioceramics material that is used for the regeneration of bone is hydroxyapatite (HA) [19–21].

Hydroxyapatite (HA) is an important class of material belonging to the calcium phosphate ceramic group which is also applied for regenerative bone surgeries. Normal human bone is mainly comprised of 69 weight% mineral apatite, 22 weight % organic component and 9 weight % water and the mineral components of the bone were formularized as calcium hydroxyapatite, which contains irregularly shaped particles of size ranges from 30 to 45 nm length and width and an average of 5 nm thickness [22].

HA with the general formula of (Ca 10(PO4)6(OH) 2) contains calcium phosphate in ratio of 1.67, that is similar to bone. HA is the stable form of calcium phosphate-based materials, which is less soluble. It contains only calcium and phosphate, so it does not cause any tissue inflammation, and is biocompatible and HA is commonly used for orthopedic, dental, and maxillofacial applications, also as a covering material for metal implants or as a bone filler [23, 24].

In daily practice, dentists encounter alveolar bone loss and the reasons include extraction, tumor surgery, or periodontitis. The resultant bone defect hampers not only for prosthetic reconstruction but also has an esthetic effect. Due to this, bone surgeries are usually performed to regenerate the lost bone and restore the alveolar ridge contour. Taking all this into consideration alveolar bone regeneration has a role in all aspects of dentistry [25–27].

Dennissen et al. which was the primary study in performing HA in over denture and submerging root therapy in vital tooth for preserving the bulk of the alveolar ridge for better retention of prostheses [28].

John W. Frame Hydroxyapatite have excellent biocompatibility, tolerated by the hard and soft tissues of the mouth and jaws, a great potential for the future. Paper reviewed the material in its physical form in both porous and solid structure and its behavior in relation to its biological effect in various sites noted for implant placement, and its technique of surgery. The known controversies and doubtsabiut the material is mainly regarding alveolar ridge augmentation [29].

Nurul Saadah Razali Alveolar ridge loss is a physiologic consequence of extraction. This event causes feasibility of implant placement, prosthetic rehabilitation and esthetic outcome. An attempt to minimize the shrinkage of the alveolar bone, socket preservation was launched to intercede with the natural process by providing a scaffold with antibacterial and regenerative properties. For decades, hydroxyapatites (HA) used as one among biomaterials used for socket preservation treatments and it was considered as biocompatible and osteoconductive [30].

Anne Handrini Dewi Determined and analyzed the potential use of HA as a substitute of bone for alveolar bone regeneration procedures. The application of HA as bone substitute intervene the healing process [31].

Niranjan Ramesh Hydroxyapatite (HA) is a bioceramic biomaterial that copies the mineral composition of bones and teeth. HA, was commonly made via various techniques in previous years, and it is found to have excellent bioactivity, osteoconductivity, and biocompatibility. HA has been used in combination with polymers in the form of bio composite implants to improve the mechanical properties and it also enhances its activity by exploiting the effects of both HA and the polymer involved in making the biocomposite [32].

Graig D. Brown A newly developed hydroxyapatite cement helps to promote regenaration of bone in craniofacial defects and was assessed to determine its potential in treating osseous defects. HAC appears to be sufficiently structurally stable for reconstruction and augmentation of non-stress-bearing portions osseous defects [33].

Yukna RA Used HA graft material shows more clinical benefits in majority of patients with extensive periodontal defects along with open flap debridement [34].

Aparna Singh HA in conjunction with resorbable collagen membrane is used as an acceptable alternative to autogenous block graft and non-resorbable membrane for treating compromised alveolar ridge deficiencies [35].

4. Applications of hydroxyapatite for regeneration of tooth structures

Regenerative dentistry a branch of regenerative medicine that emphasis on oro-dental pathologies inclusive of bone defects such as periodontitis and alveolar bone resorption and tooth destructive disease like dental carries and pulpal necrosis [36]. All these localized skeletal ailments directly influence the quality of life of patients and healthcare resources. In order to address these aliments effectively, targeted therapies towards regeneration of both tooth and bone [36, 37].

The current treatment methods consist of replacing the lost structure with direct and indirect synthetic restorative materials. In more severe cases of dental caries or traumatic incidents, dental pulp can be compromised in reversible or irreversible inflammatory responses or pulp necrosis. Regenerative endodontics includes biological procedures to replace damaged dentin or root structures as well as pulp-dentin complex cells. Pulp capping and dentin regeneration using current biomaterials have notable limitations [36]. Severe inflammatory reactions induced by the synthetic capping materials are the major drawbacks in this methodology that can result in therapy failure. To address these limitations, research in dentistry continues to bring more decisive and reliable methods. In this way, establishing novel regenerative approaches and regeneration of dentine –pulp complex is the mainstay [37, 38].

Dental pulp regeneration requires the embodiment of a scaffold conducive with the regeneration of the pulp-dentin complex. ECM-derived proteins and or other natural resources can be employed as natural scaffolds for tooth regeneration. These biological materials can be easily engineered for production of a variety of polymeric and composite scaffolds [38]. HA, a glycosaminoglycans in the extracellular matrix, can enhance cellular metabolism and mineralization in hydrogel form, as natural platform for treating dentin/pulp complex in presence of human DPSCs (Dental pulp stem cells) and apical papilla stem cells [39, 40].

Because tooth structure is complicated, complete tooth regeneration will be difficult. As the first step in tissue engineering for the tooth, regeneration of dentine or a substitute should be attempted. To reconstruct a tooth in whole or in part, adoption of a scaffold can be used to form a tooth with three-dimensional structure. Thus for the regeneration of dentine or pulp dentine complex, porous hydroxyapatite scaffold may be used. Therefore, an HA scaffold with a hollow center similar to a tooth structure was devised and used [40]. HA scaffold was effective for dentin or dentin pulp regeneration. Thus it can be a perfect choice for tooth regeneration using a hydroxyapatite cylindrical scaffold. Osteogenesis due to stem cells in the HA was also found to be excellent [40].

Hayakawa S. et al. stated that HA platforms are effective for regeneration of dentin-pulp complex. When hDFSCs seeded on Synthetic HA scaffold (ENGIpore©) and incubated for 6 weeks an intense adherence, colonization of polygonal-shaped cells to the HA platform which was similar to dentin [41].

Campodoni et al. used Mg-Hydroxyapatite on gelatin polymers which were embedded in a matrix from chitosan blend and gelatin, to create a biocompatible 3D porous composite structure. This product is similar to dentin in its architecture and chemical composition, adaptability for cells to adhere, and differentiate [42].

Hydroxyapatite can be commonly fabricated from natural sources like fishbone, coral, bovine bone, eggshell, and seashells through the calcination process. The trace ions consisting of Na+, K+, Mg2+, Sr2+, Zn2+, and Al3+, or anions like F-, Cl-, SO4 2-, and CO3 2- make HA non-stoichiometric [42]. These trace of ions, are beneficial to promote rapid bone regeneration [43].

Natural and Synthetic hydroxyapatite based materials have been preferred over allografts and autografts for hard tissue repair. Commonly associated problems with the grafts include donor site morbidity, graft shortage, graft rejection, and disease transmission [44].

HA application in orthopedics can used in restoring bone defects and augmentation of bone. The interlocked porous structure of hydroxyapatite based implant can function as an extracellular matrix, favoring tissue regeneration and cellular development. Furthermore, HA promotes firm anchorage to the surrounding tissue and the implant thus enhances the osseointegration process. The anchorage of bone for longer periods enhances the successful osseointegration, hence completely restoring the functional ability [45].

Another remarkable application of HA in tooth regeneration as HA cylinders. HA cylinders can be used for replacement of tooth. Earlier HA was used dental cements presently its also used in toothpaste [46, 47].

Porous hydroxyapatite is an excellent biomaterial for tooth regeneration. Yoshikawa et al. [40] reported the susceptibility of HA in porous structures as a platform for tooth regeneration [48].

The another application of HA is in drug delivery system. The high-binding affinity and natural porous structure of HA enhances the drug loading ability [40].

The pure form of HA is not used for hard tissue restoration because of its low and brittle load bearing capability. Hence HA is used along with polymer or in composite form for the application of hard tissue regeneration [49, 50].

In this case, the toughness, elasticity of the composite matrix which also include its compressive strength of HA ceramic phase improves the properties of HA and thus enhances the effectiveness of the scaffold when used in tooth regeneration [51].

The development of new trends lead to the fabrication of nano-HA can accelerate dentin remineralization [52]. Nano- HA provides a rich source of calcium thus it acts as shielding material against caries and dental erosion [53]. HA requires calcium hydroxide in an enormous amount and is calculated by the increased Ca/P value.

Additionally the application of nanoHA in toothpaste function as filler for the repair the sunken enamel surfaces and also favors a protective covering on the dentinal tubules that are dissolved, contributing a speedy and quick cure from tooth hypersensitivity [47, 54]. Hydoxyapatite comes with various unique kind of properties like it does not induce any inflammation or toxicity, has the capacity to chemically bond with the bone and has the property of stimulating the growth of bones [50].

5. Hydroxyapatite for dental implant surface coating

The dental implants are used as a substitution for tooth replacement and made from stainless steel, cobalt-chrome alloys or titanium. Among these materials, titanium and its alloys gained high importance due to its highest biocompatibility, mechanical properties, excellent corrosion resistance, strength and relatively low weight [55, 56].

The Ti-based implants still remain many restraints to be implanted in human body. The high modulus of elasticity of Ti compared to the bone can persuade stress shielding also the poor tribological behavior of Ti could cause severe adhesive wear and as a consequence, generate debris in the blood stream leading to bone resorption. Implant loosening may occur because of infection in the neighboring tissues and lead to implant failure [57–59].

All these limitations can be eliminated by altering the composition, morphology and surface structure making the mechanical properties intact [60].

The implant surfaces can be modified, as there is furtherance in technology and the modified implant surfaces will improve rate of osseointegration. Current modifications include plasma spraying the implant surfaces with either hydroxyapatite (HA) or titanium beads [61–64].

There are numerous reasons for coating implants with HA. The implementation of HA coatings thus alter the implant surface characteristics has been known since 1980s. Better osteoblastic activity and increased collagen levels are discern in cells growing on HA-coated Ti implants, improve bone fixation and thus increases the lifetime of metallic implants, enhancing the ingrowth of mineralized tissue improved the biological fixation, bioactivity, and biocompatibility of dental implants. Thus, it is concluded that the HA coatings on metallic implants would enhance osseointegration and thus decreasing the time from implant insertion to final reconstruction.

6. Ha coating methodology

The application of apatite coatings on dental implants is a favored surface modification. HA and fluorapatite are incompetent to be used as implants, as they are brittle in nature. Therefore, load–bearing implants have been coated with HA and Fluor apatite to enhance earlier osseointegration. Various techniques are:

1. Sol–gel coating.

2. Plasma spraying.

3. Biomimetic deposition.

4. Electrochemical deposition.
5. Electrophoretic deposition.
6. Ion sputtering
7. Ion plating.
8. Ion implantation
9. Ion-beam-associated deposition
10. Super-high-speed (SHS) blasting process
11. Dip coating

6.1 Sol–gel coating

6.1.1 Preparation of hydroxyapatite sol

For preparation of sol-gel HAp coating, a blend of calcium and phosphorus precursors are used for preparation of sol with addition of solvents like ethanol and water.

Table 4 shows the commonly used precursors and solvents for the preparation of hydroxyapatite.

6.2 Plasma spraying (PS)

In PS technology it uses a device to melt and deposit a coating material at a high velocity. A direct-current electric arc created by a high current, low voltage electrical

	Precursor	Solvent
Ca precursors	• Calcium acetate monohydrate Calcium nitrate tetrahydrate • Calcium nitrate tetrahydrate Calcium nitrate tetrahydrate calcium chloride	• Water and 1,2-ethanediol • Water • Ethanol • Water and ethanol • Water
P precursors	• Phosphoric acid • Ammonium phosphate dibasic • Triethylphosphite • Triethylphosphite • Trimethyl phosphate • Phosphorus pentoxide • diammonium hydrogen orthophosphate • Trisodium phosphate	• Water • Water • Water and ethanol • Ethanol • Water • Water

Table 4.
Precursors and solvents of HA [65].

discharge between two electrodes produces a plasma flame. The arc super heats a carrier gas stream that contains the molten HA powder. The HA is deposited on the implant by the plasma flame. Adherence of the HA to titanium is mechanical and can be promoted by a roughened substrate surface [66].

Chen et al. determined functionally graded HA/Ti composite coatings had superior mechanical properties over monolithic HA coatings. He concluded that incorporating titanium to HA coating would significantly improve the bond strength of the PS coating. PS heat treatment affects the HA coating phase by increasing crystallinity [67].

6.3 Biomimetic deposition

Bone regeneration is a biological process, and precipitation of ions from solution to form apatite can be considered. An artificial body fluid with ion concentration similar to human blood plasma is used to form biomimetic apatite [68, 69]. This is a classical method to test the bioactivity of material and, apatite formed on the surface of the material can be considered as bioactive [70].

6.4 Electrochemical deposition (ECD)

Electrochemical Deposition-A rapid and excellent method, gives excellent control of the coating material's thickness, uniformity, crystallinity, and stoichiometry. The process temperature of ECD is less compared to the plasma spray method. This method is typically used to coat hydroxyapatite (HAp, $Ca_5(PO_4)_3OH$), which is a commonly used biomaterial for bone implants. HAp is a intrinsically occurring mineral form calcium phosphate (CaP) family [71]. Therefore, HAp modification using ECD method on Ti–6Al–4 V surface have favorable results for osteoconduction. An ECD with optimized redox voltage on implant enhance the osseointegration process. This technique could have promising clinical applications to amplify the healing process and success rates of dental implantation.

6.5 Electrophoresis deposition (EPD)

EPD is a process by which, colloidal particles such as HA nano particles are suspended in a liquid medium drift under the power of an electric field which are deposited onto a counter charged electrode. Pressure is concurrently applied to HA nano particles against the electrode. The coating is formed by pressure exerted by the potential difference between the electrodes [72].

EPD are currently being used due to its low cost, easy methodology, capable of producing coatings of variable thicknesses, high deposition rate, formation of highly crystalline deposits with low residual stresses [73]. EPD can produce HA coatings ranging from <1 micron to >500 microns thick [74]. Surface patterns created on the EPD cathode create a patterned HA coating on an implant substrate to change surface topography and enhance osseointegration [75].

6.6 Ion sputtering

Electron beam evaporation and magnetron sputtering techniques are used to deposit hydroxyapatite Nano coatings, to optimize the deposition conditions and so achieve desired properties. The easy replica for ion sputtering is the diode plasma, having a pair of planar electrodes, an anode and a cathode, inside a vacuum system. Another type of sputtering employs radio frequency (RF) diodes that operate at high frequency [76]. Surface characteristics are essential because of its role in enhancing osseointegration.

6.7 Ion plating

Periimplantitis, which is a bacterial induced infection on dental implant materials in human mouth, is one kind of biomaterial centered infection. Periimplantitis is responsible for losing the bony support of the bioimplants, which may cause great damage to the patient. Bacterial adhesion resistant surfaces, multiple arc ion plating methodology, plasma nitriding are used to fabricate Ti nitride coatings on commercial pure titanium used as dental implant materials [77].

6.8 Ion implantation

Into Ti6Al4V dental implants ion implantation using CO remarkably enhanced the osseointegrationin terms of the bone–implant contact, compared to the untreated dental implants. Ion implantation treatments were carried out using a Danfysik high-current implanter Model 1090. Then the samples were ultrasonically degreased and cleaned preceding to any treatment, which were performed using gaseous precursors in a Chord is ion source [78] Chord is ion source is a filament driven ion source with a small plasma chamber designed for production of singly-charged ions.

6.9 Ion-beam-associated deposition of the HA coating

On Ti-based alloy, using ion-beam-assisted deposition an HA layer can be coated. The deposition methods composed of an electron beam vaporizing a pure hydroxyapatite target.

Argon ion beam was focused on the metal substrate for deposition. The deposited layers were amorphous. The bond strength between the layers can be increased with increasing current.

The dissolution rate in a physiological saline solution decreased remarkably. These enhancements were attributed to an increase in the Ca/P ratio of the layer [79].

With ion-beam assistance, the Ca/P ratio of the layer increased apparently due to the high sputtering rate of P compared to that of Ca from the layer being coated.

7. Super-high-speed (SHS) blasting process

Super-high-speed (SHS) blasting process is a novel method to increase the bond strength between coating layer and implant surface so as to stop exfoliation of weakly layered HA from the titanium surface. An evenly layered micron-thick HA layer could maintain micro texture of the implant surface. The coating showed increased bond strength and magnificent wettability properties [80].

7.1 Dip coating

Hydroxyapatitesol was coated onto titanium rods by a dip coating method. An ultrasonic homogenizer was used for the preparation of HA sols by dispersing HA crystals less than 100 nm length in distilled water or physiological salt solution.

Homogeneity of the surface of the HA coated titanium rods were determined by scanning electron microscopy (SEM). Tuantuan Li [79] in his study found out, after implantation of uncoated and HA dip coated titanium rods in dog femurs, new bone formation was seen only over the coated material. The bonding strength of HA coated rod was found to be increased after 4 week's of implantation, as determined by pull-out testing [79]. The dip coated titanium presented remarkable biocompatibility in bone replacement applications [71].

8. Interactions at the HA coatings-tissue interface

The cellular response at the HA coated implant and tissue interface be contingent on the proteins and bio fluid adsorbed onto the surfaces. The implant surface may release ions into the bio fluid, which in turn react with proteins, water and other constituents of the bio fluid, causing surface remodeling [80, 81]. Thus, the surface quality of dental implant and its interactions with constituents of the bio fluid are critical in determining the nature and degree of cellular behavior, especially attachment and proliferation. According to Kasemo et al. [82] the biomaterial/tissue interactions occur within a narrow interfacial zone of less than 1 nm, and these initial interfacial interactions determine the initial bony attachment [82]. Besides the release of ions, surface energy of the biomaterials also affects the initial cellular contact. 108–111 Non identical materials possess distinct surface energies. Surface energy can provide a primary indicator of potential cellular adhesion and implant surface biocompatibility [83–86]. It has been observed that materials with critical surface tensions of 20 to 30 dynes/cm exhibit minimal cell adhesion, whereas materials with critical surface tensions above this range have greater degree of bio adhesion. 114 With CaP coatings of different crystallite size, there was no significant difference in the critical surface tension [87]. Biomolecules in the biological fluids continuously adsorb on the implant surfaces are vital for controlling cellular responses. Also changes in protein conformation after adsorption on biomaterials surfaces may occur and conformational changes are suggested to elicit differences in cellular response between different biomaterials (**Table 5**) [88, 89].

9. Advances in nanoparticle incoorporated hydroxyapatite

The fundamental base of the enamel unit is HA particle, size of 20 to 40 nm. The proteins are almost degraded when the enamel reaches its evolvement. This leads to the crystallization of apatite; hence the enamel cannot be biologically remodeled [95].

Hydroxyapatite has poor ability to repair fibrous connective tissue surrounding the granules, at the same time, the porosity, surface geometry and surface chemical properties of traditional hydroxyapatite scaffolds restrict the application themselves, especially to alveolar bone repair [96].

The nano-HA formed has been found to own analogous morphology, structure, and crystallinity as a biological apatite. When compared with larger HA, nano HA constitutes good biocompatibility, nontoxicity and also having higher resorption rate [97].

Nano-HA is the ideal treatment option for treating bone defects caused by trauma or surgery. While macroscale hydroxyapatite particles or blocks have long been used to treat bone abnormalities, nanoscale hydroxyapatite particles recently been

Study/year	Author	Study description	Study arms	Results
In Vivo and In Vitro Analyses of Titanium-Hydroxyapatite Functionally Graded Material for Dental Implants. (2021). PMID: 34036104 [90]	Wang X, Wan C, Feng X, Zhao F, Wang H	Fabrication of atitanium-hydroxyapatite (Ti-HA) functionally graded material (FGM) with superior mechanical and biological properties for dental implantation.	• Ti group • Ti-HA group	• The ALP and TGF-β1 levels were slightly increased. The transcript value of ALP and TGF-βRI were high in the Ti-HA groups • TGF-βRII showed no obvious increase. • The BIC bone-implant contact (BIC) and bone volume over total volume (BV/TV) did not exhibit significant differences between the Ti and Ti-HA FGM groups (P = 0.0504). BV/TV showed the Ti-HA FGM group had better osteogenesis (P = 0.04). • Ti-HA
Induction Plasma Sprayed Nano Hydroxyapatite Coatings on Titanium for Orthopedic and Dental Implants (2011). PMID: 21552358 [91]	Mangal Roy, Amit Bandyopadhyay, Susmita Bose	Preparation of a highly crystalline nano hydroxyapatite (HA) coating on commercially pure titanium(Cp-Ti) using coupled radio frequency(RF) plasma spray	HA coatings were prepared on Ti using normal and supersonic plasma nozzles at different plate powers and working distances.	X-ray diffraction and Fourier transformed infrared spectroscopic analysis revealed the normal plasma nozzle lead to enhanced phase decomposition, increased amorphous calcium phosphate (ACP) phase formation, and serious dehydroxylation of HA. Where as coatings utilized using supersonic nozzle hold on to the crystallinity and phase purity of HA Microstructural properties,adhesive bond strengths,cytotoxicity of HA coatings showed better osteoblast formation and early implant–tissue integration
Aerosol deposition of hydroxyapatite and 4-hexylresorcinol coatings on titanium alloys for dental implants (2011). PMID: 21821331 [92]	Kim SG, Hahn BD, Park DS, Lee YC, Choi EJ, Chae WS, Baek DH, Choi JY	Aerosol deposition is a newertechnique.4-Hexylresorcinol (4-HR) is an antiseptic. The influence of the 4-HR component of HA coatings on titanium surfaces was studied in vitro and in vivo	• Group A HA • Group B HA+ 4-HR coating	MG63 cells attachement, increased osteocalcin expression and alkaline phosphatase activity, higher reverse torque value higher in HA 4-HR group. Histologic analysis, ossteogenesis value and bone implant contact value were significantly higher in the HA,4-HR group 8 weeks after surgery.

Study/year	Author	Study description	Study arms	Results
Hydroxyapatite-based composite for dental implants: an in vivo removal torque experiment.(2002). PMID: 2418015 [93]	Young-Min Kong 1, Dong-Hwan Kim, Hyoun-Ee Kim, Seong-JooHeo, Jai-Young Koak	Screw-shaped dental implants were fabricated from commercially pure Ti (c.p. Ti) The HA-based composites were made by mixing HA with Al(2) O(3)-coated ZrO(2) powders. The mechanical properties increased by a factor of 3. Reversed torque to loosen the implants in vivo was measured to estimate the osteointegration.	Group A c.p. Ti Group B HA-based composite implants	The composite implants 2-times-higher removal torque to the Ti implants (ANOVA, $p < 0.05$),
The correlation between osseointegration and bonding strength at the bone-implant interface: In-vivo & ex-vivo investigations on HA and HA/Ti coatings (2022). PMID: 36162145 [94]	Ghadami F, Amani Hamedani M, Rouhi G, Saber-Samandari S, Mehdi Dehghan M, Mashhadi-Abbas F Farzad-Mohajeri S,	The study analyzed the effects of HA and HA/Ti coatings on osseointegration,bonding strength at bone-implant interface.	Three groups 1) (CP-Ti) rods Uncoated commercial pure titanium 2) HAcoated CP-Ti rods, and 3) Composite of 50%wt HA + 50%wt Ti coated CP-Ti rods.	Pull-out tests showed that the ultimate strength of HA and HA/Ti coatings were significantly greater than the uncoated samples ($P < 0.05$). Histological assessment showed significantly improved osseointegration of HA/Ti composite coatings than with HA coatings ($P < 0.05$)

Table 5.
In vitro and in vivo studies with HA -coated dental implant surfaces.

clinically introduced in an injectable form. When combined with stem cells or growth factors and placed on a scaffold, nano-HA can be used in tissue engineering and bone or cementum regeneration. It can help with oral surgeries like cleft lip and palate repair and periodontal procedures [98]. Composites containing nano-HA are used to fill the alveolar socket and reduce alveolar bone loss immediately after extraction because they can recreate the bone structure and environment while maintaining the bone's flexibility and resistance [99].

There are various studies demonstrating applications of nanohydroxyapatite in periodontics. Lowe et al. [100] concluded that chitosan nano-HA-fucoidan scaffold has high biocompatibility and mineralization and also that the composite membrane exhibited a applicable micro architecture for cell growth and nutrient supplementation. Lee et al. [101] found out that reduced graphene oxide/HA nanocomposites accelerated bone regeneration and stimulated osteogenesis. Uysal et al. [102] evaluated the efficacy of treating periodontitis using subgingivalnano-hydroxyapatite powder with an air abrasion device combined with scaling and root planning and found that it improved clinical periodontal parameters more than scaling and root planning alone as it enhances clot adhesion to the surfaces of tooth by improving surface wettability.

The widespread application of HA in implants is due to its bioactive characteristics, which aid in the production of new bone, improve tissue integration, and speed up the healing process. As a result, it's being used to convert metallic implants' smooth, harsh surfaces into a more biocompatible, porous environment similar to hard tissues. Nano-HA is the most often employed coating material for titanium and stainless-steel implants, offering benefits such as improved bone bonding and new bone genesis, as well as improved bone-to-implant contact [103]. Another benefit of employing nano-HA as a coating for dental implants is its capacity to prevent bacterial growth, including both Gram-positive and -negative bacteria. Furthermore, implants coated with a small layer of nano-HA had a lower inflammatory response, as HA is a modulator for monocytes and macrophages, which are responsible for the early inflammatory response. Several investigations have demonstrated that, because of its chemical and chrystallographic affinity for the inorganic components of bone, this substance is capable of establishing chemical linkages and ensuring a faster integration of the implants with the bone and surrounding tissue [104]. As grafting materials in relation to dental implants, alloplast materials containing nano-HA are employed. They promote bone repair by enhancing angiogenesis and consequently having a high porosity. Because of the quicker bone growth, an earlier implant placement is permitted, with these materials having a 4-month healing period [105].

Nanohydroxyapatite in toothpaste, in particular, has been demonstrated in studies to promote remineralization and the hardness of dental enamel and dentine. This is owing to the nano-hydroxyapatite particles' incredibly small size, which allows them to easily enter and interact with sub-micrometer and nanometrescale acidic erosion damage on tooth surfaces (white spots). Calcium and phosphate ions are liberated from the nano-hydroxyapatite particles during the contact. The liberated ions enter the enamel rods and crystallize into apatite [106]. As a result, re-mineralization and restoration of the enamel surfaces occur. Despite the fact that nano particles can penetrate dental porosities, they can form a protective layer on the tooth's surface. Nano-HA is even used in sports drinks to reduce the impact on teeth. Acidic drinks increase tooth surface degradation.

Several studies have also demonstrated that using nano-hydroxyapatite in dental products can reduce bacterial colonization of tooth surfaces and dentine hypersensitivity. Studies have also indicated that calcium phosphate-based materials can be used to repair or remineralize missing, damaged, or eroded tooth enamel. HA-based materials, in particular, are commonly employed to remedy surface issues like as discolouration, voids, and chips. HA has been employed as filler for strengthening GICs and restorative resin composites on both a micro- and nano-scale [107]. Nano-HA is utilized to remineralize dentin and enamel that has been compromised by caries. The hard tissue loses mineral ions due to acid assault from bacterial metabolism in early-stage caries, while the collagen network is unharmed. The endeavor to remineralize this organic scaffold is realized by the use of nanoparticles (nano-HA, bioactive glass), which act as either direct replacements for final minerals or as a carrier for lost ions during caries assault [108].

Bleaching methods generate reactive oxygen species, which penetrate the enamel and reach the dentin, breaking organic molecules and processing lighter and clearer substances. The most common bleaching chemical is hydrogen peroxide, which has a concentration of 30–35% in a gel product. The gel is loaded with remineralizing chemicals such as fluoride calcium and hydroxyapatite in nano form to reduce hypersensitivity following bleaching, which can occur in up to 70% of bleached patients. The bleaching agent can permeate the enamel through microscopic surface flaws and beneath pores, causing sensitivity. Nano-HA paste can correct these minor enamel flaws, preventing the sensory reaction [109].

Nanomaterials can have a harmful impact on human health if they are present in the environment since their entry into the body is enabled by exposure and subsequent absorption through the skin, digestive tract, and lungs. Ingestion of nanoparticles in dental products during or after treatment; inhaling of aerosols created from nanomaterial-based composites during drilling; and direct interaction between nanomaterials and cellular tissues in the oral cavity can all result in exposure and potential harm [110]. Nanomaterials may easily interact with cell constituents such as DNA molecules, proteins, and intracellular components, which is important. It's challenging to foresee and comprehend these interaction mechanisms, elimination pathways, and immunological responses. This ambiguity stems from the fact that different nanomaterials of the same material behave differently in different biological tissues. Coatings, for example, can alter the size range, surface charge, and surface chemistry of nanomaterials in relation to cellular tissues [111].

Smart nanomaterials that aid in healing, stimulate cellular regeneration, and help in osseointegration of bioactive dental implants are now being researched. These new technologies, however, are not without their own set of problems. For example, designing a low-cost, mass-produced nano-robotic system that can perform their intended duties is a heavy task. There's also a demand for smart nanomaterials, protocols, and nano-devices that can give disease monitoring, diagnosis, prevention, and treatment techniques that are tailored to particular individuals.

10. Future perspectives

New dental products are still in high demand, both scientifically and commercially. There is currently no one solution that satisfies all of the required qualities and standards for preventative and restorative applications. The most successful technique of delivering beneficial outcomes for patients, however, is regarded to be breakthroughs in nanotechnology-based strategies for generating new products. Several active research fields are now being studied. Colloidal liquids containing millions of active nanometer scale robots might be delivered into the oral cavity to shut down certain nerves, for example, to lessen anxiety and provide greater patient comfort during dental treatments [112].

The practitioner sends the nano-robots to specific tooth positions or soft tissues once they have entered the oral canal. The nano-robots then travel into tissue structures, shutting off the sensitivity of specific nerves. The practitioner then instructs the nano-robots to restore nerve sensitivity and leave the tissues following the dental surgery. Orthodontic nano-robots could also be utilized to remodel periodontal tissues and allow painless tooth straightening, rotation, and repositioning in minutes to hours. Nano-robotic dentifrices, on the other hand, might be utilized to carry and distribute toothpastes or mouthwashes that break down organic matter or oral bacteria into harmless by-products. Nano-robots could also be utilized to administer antibiotics and medications (nano-encapsulation). While nano-sensors/robots could be used to detect and identify dangerous elements to aid in the diagnosis and treatment of diseases, thereby improving patient well-being [113].

Furthermore, recent research has shown that high-strength nanoparticles can be engineered into dental polymers to improve their strength and durability. For example, dental polymer reinforced with graphene gold nanoparticles increased mechanical characteristics, encouraged tissue formation when graphene oxide was implanted to collagen scaffold, and improved physicochemical and surface properties when graphene oxide was implanted to collagen scaffold. Carbon nanotubes and Boron Nitride nanoplatelets have also sparked interest among scientists as a viable biomaterial for dental applications. A recent study found that Boron Nitride nanoplatelets reinforcement improved the strength and fracture toughness of zirconia composites. However, conflicting investigations have demonstrated that carbon nanotubes have both cytotoxic and non-cytotoxic qualities, sparking a discussion about its possible application as a bioceramic material. As a result, bio-kinetics and organ toxicity are crucial in determining the quantitative risk of using these high-strength nanomaterials.

Furthermore, smart nanomaterials that aid in healing, stimulate cellular regeneration, and osseointegration of bioactive dental implants are now being researched. These new technologies, however, are not without their own set of problems. For example, designing low-cost, mass-produced nano-robotic systems that can perform their intended duties. There's also a demand for smart nanomaterials, protocols, and nano-devices that can give disease monitoring, diagnosis, prevention, and treatment techniques that are tailored to particular individuals.

11. Conclusion

Hydroxyapatite is biocompatible material that provides cell adhesion & proliferation. It is used as a carrier & a loading agent in the controlled release and delivery of drugs. Also used as a coating materials on orthopedic implant, because of chemical resemblance to the mineral component of mammal bone and hard tissues. Advances related to varieties of methods of synthesis of HAp, as well as knowledge and Applications of Hydroxyapatite.

HAp is generally used to treat bone and periodontal defects, alveolar ridge, as dental materials, middle ear implants, tissue engineering systems and bioactive coatings on metallic osseous implants. Recent studies also suggest that HAp particles impede the progression of cancer cells.

Due to its structural fragility, a great demand for the development of efficient, simple and low-cost methods. HAp has limited applications when the bone defect to be repaired is in anatomical regions that are under constant tension. Thus, researchers have been directing studies in obtaining materials having superior properties.

As a replacement, HAp is used with other materials, increasing its applicability and efficiency for treatment of tissues. This shows a promising methodology and high potential for the development of scaffolds.

The development of optimal bone supports, coatings and release systems are a challenge for the engineering of bone tissue. It is a requisite to study the development and applicability in different anatomical sites to improve mechanical and biological aspects of HAp-based implants and to optimize their safety and efficiency. However, the prospects of novel biomaterials such as HAp in biomedical fields definitely depend upon the advancement of our knowledge, not only of the material, but also its interactions with specific bio-molecules, cells, and tissues.

Author details

Prameetha George Ittycheria[1*], Thomas George[1], Mathew John[2], G. Meenu[1], Vimal Thomas[1], S. Aswathy[2], Rene Kuriakose[1] and Jerin Thomas[1]

1 Department of Periodontology and Implantology, Pushpagiri College of Dental Sciences, Pathanamthitta, Kerala, India

2 Department of Periodontology and Implantology, Sri Sankara Dental College, Varkala, Kerala, India

*Address all correspondence to: prameethageorgeittycheria@gmail.com

References

[1] Bee S-L, Hamid ZAA. Characterization of chicken bone waste-derived hydroxyapatite and its functionality on chitosan membrane for guided bone regeneration. Composites Part B: Engineering. 2019;**163**:562-573

[2] Chadda H, Satapathy BK, Patnaik A, Ray AR. Mechanistic interpretations of fracture toughness and correlations to wear behavior of hydroxyapatite and silica/hydroxyapatite filled bis-GMA/TEGDMA micro/hybrid dental restorative composites. Composites Part B: Engineering. 2017;**130**:132-146

[3] AbouAitah K, Stefanek A, Higazy IM, Janczewska M, Swiderska-Sroda A, Chodara A, et al. Effective targeting of colon cancer cells with piperine natural anticancer prodrug using functionalized clusters of hydroxyapatite nanoparticles. Pharmaceutics. 2020;**12**(1):28

[4] Bossu M, Saccucci M, Salucci A, Di Giorgio G, Bruni E, Uccelletti D, et al. Enamel remineralization and repair results of biomimetic hydroxyapatite toothpaste on deciduous teeth: An effective option to fluoride toothpaste. Journal of Nanbiotechnology. 2019;**17**(1):17

[5] Shibui T, Yajima T, Irie K, Ochi M, Sakakura Y. Architecture of connective tissue regenerated by enamel matrix derivative around hydroxyapatite implanted into tooth extraction sockets in the rat maxilla. Anatomical Science International. 2020;**95**(3):334-341

[6] Haugen H, Lyngstadaas S, Rossi F, Perale G. Bone grafts: Which is the ideal biomaterial? Journal of Clinical Periodontology. 2019;**46**:92-102

[7] Brydone AS, Meek D, Maclaine S. Bone grafting, orthopaedic biomaterials, and the clinical need for bone engineering. Proceedings of the Institution of Mechanical Engineers. Part H. 2010;**224**:1329-1343

[8] Laurencin C, Khan Y, El-Amin S. Bone graft substitutes. Expert Review of Medical Devices. 2006;**3**(1):49-57

[9] Nabers CL, O'Leary TJ. Autogenous bone transplant in the treatment of osseus defects. Journal of Periodontology. 1965;**36**:5-14

[10] Arrington ED, Smith WJ, Chambers HG, Bucknell AL, Davino NA. Complications of iliac crest bone graft harvesting. Clinical Orthopaedics and Related Research. 1996;**329**:300-309

[11] Beaman F, Bancroft L, Peterson J, Kransdorf M, Menke D, DeOrio J. Imaging characteristics of bone graft materials. Radiographics. 2006;**26**(2):373-388

[12] Bosshardt D, Sculean A. Does periodontal tissue regeneration really work? Periodontology 2000. 2009;**51**(1):208-219

[13] Oryan A, Alidadi S, Moshiri A, Maffulli N. Bone regenerative medicine: Classic options, novel strategies, and future directions. Journal of Orthopaedic Surgery and Research. 2014;**9**(1):18. DOI: 10.1186/1749-799X-9-18

[14] Yu X, Tang X, Gohil S, Laurencin C. Biomaterials for bone regenerative engineering. Advanced Healthcare Materials. 2015;**4**(9):1268-1285

[15] Dixon D, Gomillion C. Conductive scaffolds for bone tissue engineering: Current state and future outlook. Journal of Functional Biomaterials. 2021;**13**(1):1

[16] Huang X, Liu X, Shang Y, Qiao F, Chen G. Current trends in research on bone regeneration: A bibliometric analysis. BioMed Research International. 2020;**2020**:1-12

[17] Mancini L, Romandini M, Fratini A, Americo L, Panda S, Marchetti E. Biomaterials for periodontal and peri-implant regeneration. Materials. 2021;**14**(12):3319

[18] Balu SK, Andra S, Jeevanandam J, Manisha Vidyavathy S, Sampath V. Emerging marine derived nanohydroxyapatite and their composites for implant and biomedical applications. Journal of the Mechanical Behavior of Biomedical Materials. 2021;**119**:104523

[19] Carson JS, Bostrom MPG. Synthetic bone scaffolds and fracture repair. Injury-international Journal of The Care of The Injured. 2007;**3851**:533e537

[20] Supova M. Problem of hydroxyapatite dispersion in polymer matrices: A review. Journal of Materials Science. Materials in Medicine. 2009;**20**:1201e1213

[21] Ana ID, Matsuya S, Ishikawa K. Engineering of carbonate apatite bone substitute based on composition-transformation of gypsum and calcium hydroxide. Engineering. 2010;**2**(05):344e349

[22] LeGeros RZ. Calcium phosphate-based osteoinductive materials. Chemical Reviews. 2008;**108**(11):4742-4753. DOI: 10.1021/CR800427G

[23] Panda S, Biswas CK, Paul S. A comprehensive review on the preparation and application of calcium hydroxyapatite: A special focus on atomic doping methods for bone tissue engineering. Ceramics International. 2021;**47**:28122-28144

[24] Curran DJ, Fleming TJ, Towler MR, Hampshire S. Mechanical parameters of strontium doped hydroxyapatite sintered using microwave and conventional methods. Journal of the Mechanical Behavior of Biomedical Materials. 2011;**4**:2063-2073

[25] Bo€eck-Neto RJ, Gabrielli M, Lia R, Marcantonio E, Shibli JA, Marcantonio E Jr. Histomorphometrical analysis of bone formed after maxillary sinus floor augmentation by grafting with a combination of autogenous bone and demineralized freeze-dried bone allograft or hydroxyapatite. Journal of Periodontology. 2002;**73**(3):266e270

[26] Lindgren C, Hallman M, Sennerby L, Sammons R. Back-scattered electron imaging and elemental analysis of retrieved bone tissue following sinus augmentation with deproteinized bovine bone or biphasic calcium phosphate. Clinical Oral Implants Research. 2010;**21**(9):924e930

[27] Karabuda C, Ozdemir O, Tosun T, Anil A, Olgaç V. Histological and clinical evaluation of 3 different grafting materials for sinus lifting procedure based on 8 cases. Journal of Periodontology. 2001;**72**(10):1436e1442

[28] Denissen HW, de Groot K. Immediate dental root implants from synthetic dense calcium hydroxylapatite. The Journal of Prosthetic Dentistry. 1979;**42**(5):551-556. DOI: 10.1016/0022-3913(79)90253-1

[29] Frame JW. Hydroxyapatite as a biomaterial for alveolar ridge augmentation. International Journal

of Oral and Maxillofacial Surgery. 1987;**16**(6):642-655

[30] Hassan MI, Younis LT, Razali NS. The application of hydroxyapatite in socket preservation: A review of the past and current advancement. Journal of Pharmaceutical Research International. 2022:7-14

[31] Dewi AH, Ana ID. The use of hydroxyapatite bone substitute grafting for alveolar ridge preservation, sinus augmentation, and periodontal bone defect: A systematic review. Heliyon. 2018;**4**(10):e00884

[32] Ramesh N, Ratnayake J, Dias G. Calcium-based ceramic biomaterials. 2021. pp. 333-394. DOI: 10.1016/B978-0-12-818831-6.00011-2

[33] Brown GD, Mealey BL, Nummikoski PV, Bifano SL, Waldrop TC. Hydroxyapatite cement implant for regeneration of periodontal osseous defects in humans. Journal of Periodontology. 1998;**69**(2):146-157

[34] Yukna RA. Osseous defect responses to hydroxylapatite grafting versus open flap debridement. Journal of Clinical Periodontology. 1989;**16**(7):398-402

[35] Singh A, Daing A, Anand V, Dixit J. Two dimensional alveolar ridge augmentation using particulate hydroxyapatite and collagen membrane: A case report. journal of Oral Biology and Craniofacial Research. 2014;**4**(2):151-154

[36] Tran SD, Bakkar MO, Sumita Y, Kishimoto N. Regenerative dentistry in periodontics. The Saudi Dental Journal. 2019;**31**:301

[37] Hilton TJ. Keys to clinical success with pulp capping: A review of the literature. Operative Dentistry. 2009;**34**:615

[38] Almeida LDF, Babo PS, Silva CR, Rodrigues MT, Hebling J, Reis RL, et al. Hyaluronic acid hydrogels incorporating platelet lysate enhance human pulp cell proliferation and differentiation. Journal of Materials Science. Materials in Medicine. 2018;**29**:88

[39] Chrepa V, Austah O, Diogenes A. Evaluation of a commercially available hyaluronic acid hydrogel (restylane) as injectable scaffold for dental pulp regeneration: An in vitro evaluation. Journal of Endodontia. 2017;**43**:257

[40] Yoshikawa M, Tsuji N, Toda T, Ohgushi H. Osteogenic effect of hyaluronic acid sodium salt in the pores of a hydroxyapatite scaffold. Materials Science and Engineering: C. 2007;**27**:220-226

[41] Hayakawa S, Li Y, Tsuru K, Osaka A, Fujii E, Kawabata K. Preparation of nanometer scale rod array of hydroxyapatite crystal. ActaBiomater. 2009;**5**:2152-60. 22

[42] Campodoni E, Dozio SM, Panseri S, Montesi M, Tampieri A, Sandri M. Mimicking natural microenvironments: Design of 3D-aligned hybrid scaffold for dentin regeneration. Frontiers in Bioengineering and Biotechnology. 2020;**8**:836

[43] Jang CH, Cho YB, Choi CH, Jang YS, Jung WK, Lee JK. Comparision of osteoconductivity of biologic and artificial synthetic hydroxyapatite in experimental mastoid obliteration. Acta Oto-Laryngologica. 2014;**134**(3):255-259

[44] Rincón-López JA, Hermann-MuñozJA, Giraldo-BetancurAL, De Vizcaya-Ruiz A, Alvarado-Orozco JM, Muñoz-Saldaña J. Synthesis,

characterization and in vitro study of synthetic and bovine-derived hydroxyapatite ceramics: A comparison. Materials (Basel). 2018;**11**(3)

[45] Park J, Kim BJ, Hwang JY, Yoon YW, Cho HS, Kim DH, et al. In-vitro mechanical performance study of biodegradable polylactic acid/ hydroxyapatite nanocomposites for fixation medical devices. Journal of Nanoscience and Nanotechnology. 2018;**18**(2):837-841

[46] Shi P, Liu M, Fan F, Yu C, Lu W, Du M. Characterization of natural hydroxyapatite originated from fish bone and its biocompatibility with osteoblasts. Materials Science & Engineering. C, Materials for Biological Applications. 2018;**90**:706-712

[47] Ganss C, Marten J, Hara AT, Schlueter N. Toothpastes and enamel erosion/abrasion—Impact of active ingredients and the particulate fraction. Journal of Dentistry. 2016;**54**:62-67

[48] Figliuzzi MM, Giudice A, Pileggi S, Scordamaglia F, Marrelli M, Tatullo M, et al. Biomimetic hydroxyapatite used in the treatment of periodontal intrabony pockets: Clinical and radiological analysis. Annali di Stomatologia (Roma). 2016;7(1-2):16-23

[49] Lai W, Chen C, Ren X, Lee IS, Jiang G, Kong X. Hydrothermal fabrication of porous hollow hydroxyapatite microspheres for a drug delivery system. Materials Science & Engineering. C, Materials for Biological Applications. 2016;**62**:166-172

[50] Vamze J, Pilmane M, Skagers A. Biocompatibility of pure and mixed hydroxyapatite and α-tricalcium phosphate implanted in rabbit bone. Journal of Materials Science. Materials in Medicine. 2015;**26**(2):73

[51] Cheng Y, Zhao G, Liu H. Histological evaluation of collagen-hydroxyapatite composite as osseous implants in the repair of mandibular defect. Zhongguo Xiu Fu Chong Jian Wai Ke Za Zhi. 1998;**12**(2):74-76

[52] Albertini M, Fernandez-Yague M, Lázaro P, Herrero-Climent M, Rios-Santos JV, Bullon P, et al. Advances in surfaces and osseointegration in implantology. Biomimetic surfaces. Medicina Oral, Patología Oral y Cirugía Bucal. 2015;**20**(3):e316-e325

[53] Peng F, Veilleux E, Schmidt M, Wei M. Synthesis of hydroxyapatite nanoparticles with tailorable morphologies and carbonate substitutions using a wet precipitation method. Journal of Nanoscience and Nanotechnology. 2012;**12**(3):2774-2782

[54] Debnath T, Chakraborty A, Pal TK. A clinical study on the efficacy of hydroxyapatite—Bioactive glass composite granules in the management of periodontal bony defects. Journal of Indian Society of Periodontology. 2014;**18**(5):593-600

[55] Niinomi M, Nakai M, Hieda J. Development of new metallic alloys for biomedical applications. Acta Biomaterialia. 2012;**8**:3888-3903

[56] Qin L, Liu C, Yang K, Tang B. Characteristics and wear performance of borided Ti6Al4V alloy prepared by double glow plasma surface alloying. Surface and Coating Technology. 2013;**225**:92-96

[57] De Viteri VS, Fuentes E. Titanium and titanium alloys as biomaterials. In: Gegner J, editor. Tribology—Fundamentals and Advancements. Vol. 55. London, UK, London, UK: IntechOpen; 2013. pp. 561-565

[58] Wolford L. Factors to consider in joint prosthesis systems. Baylor University Medical Center Proceedings. 2006;**19**:232-238

[59] Chandra A, Ryu J, Karra P, Shrotriya P, Tvergaard V, Gaisser M, et al. Life expectancy of modular Ti6Al4V hip implants: Influence of stress and environment. Journal of the Mechanical Behavior of Biomedical Materials. 2011;**4**:1990-2001

[60] Daculsi G. History of Development and Use of the Bioceramics and Biocomposites. Cham, Switzerland: Springer International Publishing; 2016

[61] Branemark P. Osseointegration and its experimental background. The Journal of Prosthetic Dentistry. 1981;**50**:399-403

[62] Jarcho M. Calcium phosphate ceramics as hard tissue prosthetics. Clinical Orthopaedics. 1981;**157**: 259-278

[63] Jarcho M. Biomaterial aspects of calcium phosphates. Properties and applications. Dental Clinics of North America. 1986;**30**:25-47

[64] Wennerberg A, Albrektsson T, Andersson B. Design and surface characteristics ofm13 commercially available oral implant systems. The International Journal of Oral & Maxillofacial Implants. 1993;**8**:622-633

[65] Jaafar A, Hecker C, Árki P, Joseph Y. Sol-gel derived hydroxyapatite coatings for titanium implants: A review. Bioengineering. 2020;7(4):127

[66] Ong JL, Carnes DL, Bessho K. Evaluation of titanium plasma-sprayed and plasma-sprayed hydroxyapatite implants in vivo. Biomaterials. 2004;**25**(19):4601-4606

[67] Chen W, Liu Y, Courtney H, Bettenga M, Agrawal CM, Bumgardner JD, et al. In vitro anti-bacterial and biological properties of magnetron co-sputtered silver-containing hydroxyapatite coating. Biomaterials. 2006;**27**(32):5512-5517

[68] Kokubo T, Takadama H. How useful is SBF in predicting in vivo bone bioactivity? Biomaterials. 2006;**27**(15):2907-2915

[69] Uchida M, Kim HM, Kokubo T, Fujibayashi S, Nakamura T. Structural dependence of apatite formation on titania gels in a simulated body fluid. Journal of Biomedical Materials Research. Part A. 2003;**64**(1):164-170

[70] Lee K, Park M, Kim HM, Lim YJ, Chun HJ, Kim H. Ceramic bioactivity: progresses, challenges and perspectives. Biomedical Materials. 2006;**2006**(1)

[71] Huang HY, Manga YB, Huang W-N, Lin C-K, Tseng C-L, Huang H-M, et al. Effect of hydroxyapatite formation on titanium surface with bone morphogenetic protein-2 loading through electrochemical deposition on MG-63 Cells. Materials (Basel). 2018;**11**(10):1897

[72] Rosenstock HB, Schulman JH. Models for luminescence degradation in organic solids. The Journal of Chemical Physics. 1959;**30**(1):116-125

[73] Wang Y, Zhang S, Wei K, Zhao N, Chen J, Wang X. Hydrothermal synthesis of hydroxyapatite nanopowders using cationic surfactant as a template. Materials Letters. 2006;**60**(12):1484-1487

[74] We M, Ruys AJ, Swain MV, Milthorpe BK, Sorrell CC. Hydroxyapatite-coated metals: Interfacial reactions during sintering. Journal of Materials Science. Materials in Medicine.

2005;**16**(2):101-106. DOI: 10.1007/s10856-005-5995-6

[75] Wang R, Hu YX. Patterning hydroxyapatite biocoating by electrophoretic deposition. Journal of Biomedical Materials Research. 2003;**67A**(1):270-275

[76] Choi J-M, Kim H-E, Lee's I-S. Ion-beam-assisted deposition (IBAD) of hydroxyapatite coating layer on Ti-based metal substrate. Biomaterials. 2000;**21**(5):469-473. DOI: 10.1016/S0142-9612(99)00186-6

[77] Mediaswanti K, Wen C, Ivanova EPC, Berndt C, Wang J. Sputtered hydroxyapatite Nanocoatings on novel titanium alloys for biomedical applications. In: Sieniawski J, Ziaja W, editors. Titanium Alloys—Advances in Properties Control. London: IntechOpen; 2013

[78] Lin N, Huang X, Zou J, Zhang X, Qin L, Fan A, et al. Effects of plasma nitriding and multiple arc ion plating TiN coating on bacterial adhesion of commercial pure titanium via in vitro investigations. Surface and Coating Technology. 2012;**209**:212-215

[79] Li T, Lee J, Kobayashi T, Aoki H. Hydroxyapatite coating by dipping method, and bone bonding strength. Journal of Materials Science: Materials in Medicine. 1996;**7**:355-357

[80] Jung UW, Hwang JW, Choi DY, Hu KS, Kwon MK, Choi SH, et al. Surface characteristics of a novel hydroxyapatite-coated dental implant. Journal of Periodontal and Implant Science. 2012;**42**(2):59-63. DOI: 10.5051/jpis.2012.42.2.59

[81] McQueen D, Sundgren J-E, Lvarsson B, Lundstrom I, Af Ekenstam B, Svensson A, et al. Auger electron spectroscopic studies of titanium implants. In: Lee AJC, Albrektsson T, Branemark PI, editors. Clinical Applications of Biomaterials. New York: Wiley; 1982. pp. 179-185

[82] Kasemo B, Lausmaan J. Surface science aspects on inorganic biomaterials. CRC Critical Reviews in Biocompatibility. 1986;**2**:335-380

[83] Baier RE, Meyer AE, Akers CK, Natiella JR, Meenaghan M, Carter JM. Degradative effects of conventional steam sterilization on biomaterial surfaces. Biomaterials. 1982;**3**:241-245

[84] Baier RE, Meyer AE, Natiella JR, Carter JM. Surface properties determine bioadhesive outcomes: Methods and results. Journal of Biomedical Materials Research. 1984;**18**:337-345

[85] Baier RE, Meyer AE. Implant surface preparation. The International Journal of Oral & Maxillofacial Implants. 1988;**3**:9-20

[86] Hanker JS, Giammara BL. Biomaterials and biomedical devices. Science. 1988;**242**:885-892

[87] Ong JL, Raikar GN, Smoot TM. Properties of calcium phosphate coatings before and after exposure to simulated biological fluid. Biomaterials. 1997;**18**:1271-1275

[88] Andrade JD. Principles of protein adsorption. In: Andrade JD, editor. Surface and Interfacial Aspects of Biomedical Polymers. Vol. 2. New York: Plenum; 1985. pp. 1-80

[89] Williams RL, Williams DF. The spatial resolution of protein adsorption on surfaces of heterogeneous metallic biomaterials. Journal of Biomedical Materials Research. 1989;**23**:339-350

[90] Wang X, Wan C, Feng X, Zhao F, Wang H. In vivo and In vitro analyses of titanium-hydroxyapatite functionally graded material for dental implants. BioMed Research International. 2021;**2021**:8859945. DOI: 10.1155/2021/8859945

[91] Roy M, Bandyopadhyay A, Bose S. Induction plasma sprayed Nano hydroxyapatite coatings on titanium for orthopaedic and dental implants. Surface and Coating Technology. 2011;**205**(8-9):2785-2792. DOI: 10.1016/j.surfcoat.2010.10.042

[92] Kim SG, Hahn BD, Park DS, Lee YC, Choi EJ, Chae WS, et al. Aerosol deposition of hydroxyapatite and 4-hexylresorcinol coatings on titanium alloys for dental implants. Journal of Oral and Maxillofacial Surgery. 2011;**69**(11):e354-e363. DOI: 10.1016/j.joms.2011.06.002

[93] Kong YM, Kim DH, Kim HE, Heo SJ, Koak JY. Hydroxyapatite-based composite for dental implants: An in vivo removal torque experiment. Journal of Biomedical Materials Research. 2002;**63**(6):714-721. DOI: 10.1002/jbm.10392

[94] Ghadami F, Amani Hamedani M, Rouhi G, Saber-Samandari S, Mehdi Dehghan M, Farzad-Mohajeri S, et al. The correlation between osseointegration and bonding strength at the bone-implant interface: In-vivo & ex-vivo investigations on hydroxyapatite and hydroxyapatite/titanium coatings. Journal of Biomechanics. 2022;**144**:111310. DOI: 10.1016/j.jbiomech.2022.111310

[95] Gomes DS, Santos AMC, Neves GA, Menezes RR. A brief review on hydroxyapatite production and use in biomedicine. Cerâmica. 2019;**65**(374):282-302. DOI: 10.1590/0366-69132019653742706

[96] Mingzu D, Chen J, Liu K, Xing H, Song C. Recent advances in biomedical engineering of nano-hydroxyapatite including dentistry, cancer treatment and bone repair. Composites Part B: Engineering. 2021. DOI: 10.1016/j.compositesb.2021.108790

[97] Pagano S, Coniglio M, Valenti C, et al. Biological effects of resin monomers on oral cell populations: Descriptive analysis of literature. European Journal of Paediatric Dentistry. 2019;**20**(3):224-232. DOI: 10.23804/ejpd.2019.20.03.11

[98] Gupta D, Venugopal J, Mitra S, Giri Dev VR, Ramakrishna S. Nanostructured biocomposite substrates by electrospinning and electrospraying for the mineralization of osteoblasts. Biomaterials. 2009;**30**:2085-2094

[99] Svanborg LM, Hoffman M, Andersson M, Currie F, Kjellin P, Wennerberg A. The effect of hydroxyapatite nanocrystals on early bone formation surrounding dental implants. International Journal of Oral and Maxillofacial Surgery. 2011;**40**:308-315

[100] Lowe B, Venkatesan J, Anil S, Shim MS, Kim SK. Preparation and characterization of chitosan-natural nano hydroxyapatite-fucoidan nanocomposites for bone tissue engineering. International Journal of Biological Macromolecules. 2016;**93**(Pt B):1479-1487. DOI: 10.1016/j.ijbiomac.2016.02.054. Epub 2016 Feb 26. PMID: 26921504

[101] Lee JH, Shin YC, Lee SM, Jin OS, Kang SH, Hong SW, et al. Enhanced osteogenesis by reduced graphene oxide/hydroxyapatite nanocomposites. Scientific Reports. 2015;**5**:18833

[102] Uysal O, Ustaoğlu G, Behçet M, Albayrak O, Tunal M. Applying nano-HA

in addition to scaling and root planning increases clinical attachment gain. Journal of Periodontal and Implant Science. 2021;**51**(6):e41

[103] Masahiro Y, Takeshi U, Naoki T, Takayuki I, Kaori N, Norio H, et al. Boneintegration capability of nanopoyimorphic crystalline hydroxyapatite coated on titanium implants. International Journal of Nanomedicine. 2012;**7**:859-873

[104] Yang GL, He FM, Hu JA, Wang XX, Zhao SF. Effects of biomimetically and electrochemically deposited nano-hydroxyapatite coatings on osseointegration of porous titanium implants. Oral Surgery, Oral Medicine, Oral Pathology, Oral Radiology. 2009;**107**:782-789

[105] Dhivya S, Saravanan S, Sastry TP, Selvamurugan N. Nanohydroxyapatite-reinforced chitosan composite hydrogel for bone tissue repair in vitro and in vivo. Journal of Nanobiotechnology. 2015;**13**(40):21

[106] Marchisio O, Esposito M, Genovesi A. Salivary pH level and bacterial plaque evaluation in orthodonticpatients treated with Recaldent® products. International Journal of Dental Hygiene. 2010;**8**:232-236

[107] Cai Y, Tang R. Calcium phosphate nanoparticles in biomineralization and biomaterials. Journal of Materials Chemistry. 2008;**18**:3775-3787

[108] Li L, Pan H, Tao J, Xu X, Mao C, Gu X, et al. Repair of enamel by using hydroxyapatite nanoparticles as the building blocks. Journal of Materials Chemistry. 2008;**18**:4079-4084

[109] Pepla E, Besharat LK, Palaia G, Tenore G, Migliau G. Nano-hydroxyapatite and its applications inpreventive, restorative and regenerative dentistry: A review of literature. Annali di stomatologia (Roma). 2014;**5**:108-114

[110] Rocks SA, Pollard SJ, Dorey RA, Harrison PT, Levy LS, Handy RD, et al. Risk assessment of manufactured nanomaterials. In: Environmental and Human Health Impacts of Nanotechnology. Hoboken: Blackwell Publishing Ltd; 2009. pp. 389-421

[111] Barnard AS. Nanohazards: Knowledge is our first defence. Nature Materials. 2006;**5**:245-248

[112] Markan S, Lehl G, Kapoor S. Recent advances of nanotechnology in endodontics, conservative and preventive dentistry—A review. Journal of Dentistry and Oral Biology. 2017;**2**:1067

[113] Verma SK, Prabhat KC, Goyal L, Rani M, Jain A. A critical review of the implication of nanotechnology in modern dental practice. National Journal of Maxillofacial Surgery. 2010;**1**:41-44